LEARNING TO FALL

54-SIMM

LEARNING TO FALL

FALL

The Blessings of an Imperfect Life

PHILIP SIMMONS

Homefarm Books
Sandwich, New Hampshire

This book was printed in the United States of America.

Portions of this book have appeared previously, in somewhat
different form, in the *UU World*, the journal of the Unitarian
Universalist Association.

Homefarm Books
P.O. Box 114
Center Sandwich, NH 03227
homefarm@worldpath.net

To order additional copies of this book, contact:
Xlibris Corporation
1-888-7-XLIBRIS
www.Xlibris.com
Orders@Xlibris.com

CONTENTS

DEDICATION

For Kathryn, Aaron, and Amelia

ACKNOWLEDGEMENTS

W e tend to think of spiritual growth as an individual mat
ter, and of writing as a solitary profession, but I know
that both my journey and my writing have been shaped by
the people among whom I have lived and worked, and that
this book wouldn't have been possible without them. I've
been lucky to be a part of the challenging and nurturing religious community of the North Shore Unitarian Church of
Deerfield, Illinois, where the first portions of what would
eventually grow into this book found a welcoming audience.
I'm especially grateful to the Rev. Gary James, Tim Dirsmith,
and Greg Rodriguez for their friendship and support, and to
Wayland Rogers for the transforming power of his musician-
ship. Gil Schwartz was for several crucial years my guide
through the thickets of spiritual understanding, and contrib-
uted substantially to my knowledge of Jewish, Buddhist, and
Hindu traditions and texts. Lake Forest College generously
supported my professional and personal growth during the
nine years I spent as an active member of its faculty; I'm
grateful to the College as well for the sabbatical leave during
which much of this book was written, and to Ron Miller and
Cathy Benton of the Religion department for sharing their
knowledge of both Eastern and Western religious traditions.

I'm grateful to the folks at the *UU World*—Tom Stites, Amy Hoffman, and especially David Reich—for their consistent support of my work, and to David Reich, again, for his sensitive and intelligent editing of this manuscript. My thanks go to my agent, Bob Markel, for his enthusiasm and savvy and heart, and to publicist Jodee Blanco, whose spirited work on this project honors the memory of Joni Grenier. I'm grateful for the big hearts and inquiring minds I've found at the Starr King Unitarian Universalist Fellowship in Plymouth, New Hampshire, and especially for the caring work of its minister, the Rev. Arthur Vaeni. Peggy Johnson, of Wonalancet and the world, has been my musical collaborator at many church services and other events where I have performed readings from this book, has provided a listening ear as I talked my way through its writing, and has turned her skills to the design of its cover. For her unstinting support and friendship I am immeasurably grateful. I want to thank all my friends in Sandwich, New Hampshire, who have encouraged me during the writing of this book, including all those who have attended my various readings, talks, and church services. The Revs. Mark Henderson, John Woolverton, and David Blackshear have generously shared their religious perspectives and aided my study of biblical texts. Special thanks to Derek Marshall, Frances Strayer, Jan Sutherland, and all the members of FOPAK for bringing encouragement, friendship, and good meals to my family and me during trying times.

My parents, Mary and Alan Simmons, had the imagination and pluck to bring our family to New Hampshire in the first place, and I'm thankful for their daily presence in my life and the lives of my children. As for my children, Aaron and Amelia, there are many days when they alone seem to make my life possible, and certainly I couldn't have written this book without their daily instruction in the art of living fully. My deepest debt of gratitude goes to my wife and soul mate,

Kathryn Field, who sustains me each day with her love and care, and without whom this book and much of what has been most precious in my life would not have come to pass.

FOREWORD

This book is for everyone who has lived long enough to discover that life is both more and less than we hoped for. We've known earth's pleasures: sunlight on a freshly mowed lawn, leaves trembling with rain, a child's laugh, the sight of a lover stepping from the bath. We've also seen marriages sour and careers crash, we've seen children lost to illness and accident. But beyond the dualities of feast and famine we've glimpsed something else: the blessings shaken out of an imperfect life like fruit from a blighted tree. We've known the dark woods, but also the moon. This book is for those ready to embrace this third way, the way *through* loss to a wholeness, richness, and depth we had never before envisioned.

We're stubborn creatures, and it takes a shock to make us see our lives afresh. In my case the shock was the news, when I was just 35 years old, that I had the fatal condition known as ALS, or Lou Gehrig's disease, and would likely be dead within a few years. By now—more than seven years later—I've outlived those predictions and also the sense that my predicament is so unusual. Life, after all, is a terminal condition. At some point we all confront the fact that each of us, each individual soul is, as the poet William Butler Yeats says, "fastened to a dying animal." We're all engaged in the business of dying, whether consciously or not, slowly or not. For me, knowing that my days are numbered has meant the chance to ask with new urgency the sorts of questions most of us avoid: everything from "What is my life's true purpose?" to "Should I reorganize my closets?" What I've learned from asking them is that a fuller consciousness of my own mortality has been my best guide to being more fully alive.

You will bring your own experiences of loss, whether physical or emotional, to your reading of this book. You'll bring your own versions of happiness, too. Whatever need or curiosity or accident has brought you here, I hope that by reading my stories, you'll connect more deeply with your own. Just a few weeks ago, I spoke at a local church here, and though I'm not a minister I did my ministerial duty of greeting people at the church door when the service was over. Two days later, I received a note from a woman about how much my sermon had meant to her. Just as important, she wrote, had been our conversation after the service: "When I spoke to you at the door, you said, 'Praise God,' which I believe you meant not as an exclamation but as a directive. I will." Funny thing is, I never said, "Praise God." It's not the sort of thing I *would* say. But apparently it's what she needed to hear. I've learned from years of teaching college students, and from reading my writings to dozens of audiences, that people will take away from my performances whatever they most need or are most ready to receive. Often the effect has little to do with what I consciously intended. This is a humbling lesson for a teacher with a certain perspective to impart, or for a writer, whose business, after all, is controlling the responses of his or her readers.

People bring their own contexts, their particular needs and gifts and sensibilities, to the work of learning to live richly in the face of loss—work that I call "learning to fall." I'm not in the business of issuing directives, offering tips, imposing lists of spiritual dos and don'ts, or providing neat, comforting formulas. For one thing, tips and formulas take us only so far. We often deal with loss, for example, by reminding ourselves of what we still have. The man who loses his wife suddenly to cancer at age 50 is told by his friends, "You have your health, your children, your work." Such consolations help, and I have needed them often enough myself. I can't hike the high mountain ridges anymore, I tell myself, but I can take my wheelchair out on a mountain road and smell the balsam fir. It's all a matter of perspective, we like to say. (What does the snail say when riding on the turtle's back? "Whee!") But I've learned the hard way that too often the comfort provided by such thoughts resembles the brief high I get from eating chocolate; soon after, I plunge into irritability and depression. The approach I've found more helpful is also more difficult. It is born out of a paradox: that we deal most fruitfully with loss by accepting the fact that we will one day lose everything. When we learn to fall, we learn that only by letting go our grip on all that we ordinarily find most precious— our achievements, our plans, our loved ones, our very selves— can we find, ultimately, the most profound freedom. In the act of letting go of our lives, we return more fully to them. This is my book's central theme. Each essay here takes it up from a different angle and provides another lesson in the art of falling.

But I should add that when I use the word "lesson," I don't mean to suggest you should read this book for techniques or knowledge or, worse, *information.* Techniques and information are good for solving problems and fixing things, but again, that's not what I'm up to here. As I see it, we know we're truly grown up when we stop trying to fix people. About all we can really do for people is love them and treat them with kindness. That goes for ourselves, too. That goes for ourselves *especially.* I've given up on self-improvement. (I've also decided I no longer have to floss.) Fact is, my character is pretty much set, and even if I were in perfect health, I would have to accept the following truths: my desk will always be messy; I will never stop being bothered by other people's errors of grammar; I don't find badly done children's school concerts "cute"; I pick my nose; I notice beautiful women; I can't stand laziness, whether physical, moral, or intellectual; I cry during sappy father-and-son moments in movies; I will drop almost anything to watch my daughter comb her hair. For better or worse, these things are beyond fixing. Accepting ourselves means accepting the whole package, the whole sour and sweet, lovely and larcenous mess that we are.

So, too, with accepting the world, with its madness and mayhem but also its music. Right now with my weakened arms I can barely lift a Kleenex to blow my nose. But I can sit with my son as he identifies the broad-winged hawk circling over our field. This is a world I choose to remain in. We must understand what we can, and learn to dwell richly in the mystery of what we cannot. Certainly much in the world needs fixing, and there's much about the behavior of others we would like to change. But before we go fixing others, we must first accept and find compassion for ourselves. Doing so, we may begin to find that others don't need "fixing" so much as simple kindness. When we stop seeing the world as a "problem" to be solved, when instead we open our hearts to the mystery of our common suffering, we may find ourselves where we least expected to be: in a world transformed by love. If that's a directive, so be it. Reading this book, you may learn something about Buddhist philosophy or Wallace Stevens' poetry or the behavior of snapping turtles. But if my writings bring you to greater compassion for yourself and others, they will have done their work.

In polite conversation, we learn to avoid the topic of religion, which can be divisive. Wanting to avoid giving offence, it's safer, when pressed to share our views, to speak of "spirituality" rather than religion as such. But my book does deal with religious matters, and I should say something about my approach to them. So here's a story that begins like a joke: a Catholic, a Muslim, and a Buddhist, all faculty members at a small midwestern college, were leaving a lecture hall where I had given a reading from the manuscript for this book. "Sounds like Catholicism to me," said the Catholic. "No, it sounds like Sufi mysticism," said the Muslim. "No, it's Buddhism," said the Buddhist. When one of the three told me this story, I was delighted. And I could add, from my experience with other audiences, that Protestants, atheists, Jews, church dropouts, and the just plain spiritually confused have been happy to claim these writings as speaking for them, too. My approach to religion is eclectic and, I hope, inclusive. You don't need any particular background or special knowledge to read this book. You don't have to believe one thing or another. I write as a teacher and scholar of the English and American literary tradition, and as someone with a solid grounding both in my Judeo-Christian heritage—as the son of a Jewish father and a Catholic mother—and in Eastern religious traditions and practices, which I have been studying for 25 years. But most important, I write as a man—a husband, father, son, brother, and friend—who has been given an extraordinary chance to practice consciously the art of living and dying. I'm grateful for insight wherever I find it, whether in modern poetry or physics or the Koran or the Old Testament or the sayings of the Christian Desert Fathers. Of all the sources of insight available to me, I turn to religion in particular because it is with religious language that human beings have most consistently, rigorously, and powerfully explored the harrowing business of rescuing joy from heartbreak.

I also turn to humor. For the obvious reasons: diversion, relief. I could also claim health benefits, for laughter, I'm told, releases good chemicals into the brain. But more important, if we can't laugh, we can't properly be serious. Hunting for the truth about ourselves, we often resemble Elmer Fudd hunting that "wascally wabbit." The very seriousness with which we pursue truth—think of the hapless, shotgun-toting Fudd, stalking his prey—can be funny. I first learned this in college, when the Dalai Lama of Tibet came to speak to us. At the time I had only the haziest understanding of this man's importance, and I remember nothing of what he said about world peace. But I do remember his laugh. He laughed often and easily, usually at himself. Despite all he had been through—the forced occupation of his country by the Chinese, his own life in exile—he was plainly in love with the world and at peace with himself. He showed me that no one comes to self-knowledge without finding much to laugh at along the way. When I find myself getting unbearably earnest, I try to remember his example.

In my own search for peace, I've been lucky to spend time in a small woods cabin at the southern edge of New Hampshire's White Mountains, where over the past three years I've written this book. I've arranged the book's 12 essays in the order in which they were written. In them, you will see my children grow older; you will see me progress from climbing mountains to climbing into a wheelchair. You will also see that no matter how my personal circumstances change, my grounding in this place—its granite and hemlock, mosquitoes and storms, coyotes and people—remains firm and informs everything I write.

I've written this foreword during odd hours stolen from the rush of an entire busy summer, and now I find myself in late August, with the nights cool and the crickets thick in the fields. Already the first blighted leaves glow scarlet on the red maples. It's a season of fullness and sweet longings made sweeter now by the fact that I can't be sure I'll see this time of year again. Of course, none of us can name the season of his or her ending. We know only that, eventually, a particular glimpse of late afternoon's golden light filtered through green leaves will be our last. Life *is* both more and less than we hoped for, both more comic and tragic than we knew. Comedy ends in happiness, while tragedy yields wisdom. We want, I suppose, to be happily wise and wisely happy. Only then can we know the full blessings of our imperfect lives.

Sandwich, New Hampshire
August, 2000

1

LEARNING TO FALL

Because I've spent the happier parts of my life at the southern edge of New Hampshire's White Mountains, two peaks rule my imagination: Mount Washington for its sheer size, its record winds and killing weather, and Mount Chocorua for its noble profile and for the legend of the defiant Pequawket Indian chief who leaped to his death from its summit, cursing the white men who had pursued him there. I climbed Chocorua many times as a boy, and from the time of our courtship, my wife and I counted a hike to its summit as one of our annual rituals. On one such hike we made the romantic and wildly impractical decision to build a seasonal home here in New Hampshire, the place of my boyhood summers, over a thousand miles away from the Midwestern flatlands where we live and work most of the year. On the same hike, incidentally, I talked a teenage boy out of jumping off of the large angular boulder that perches just a few yards down from the summit on the east side. The boy had climbed atop the rock, about the size of a one-car garage, and then could not quite bring himself to climb down again. As he was on the point of leaping, encouraged by his friends below, I summoned my best classroom voice and said "Don't do that." I then talked him down the way he had come up. In the back of my mind I was thinking that this young man was not cut out for Chief Chocorua's fate.

Barring a miracle, I'll not climb Chocorua again. It's been almost four years since I was diagnosed with Lou Gehrig's disease, a degenerative and ultimately fatal neurological disease with no effective treatment and no cure. In that time, I've managed to finish climbing all 49 of the New Hampshire peaks above 4,000 feet, a task begun at age six with my first ascent of Mount Washington. Now, however, my legs won't go the distance, and I must content myself with the lesser triumphs of getting on my socks in the morning and making it down the stairs. On the day last summer when I began writing this essay, my wife Kathryn and our seven-year-old son Aaron were climbing Mount Washington without me. Unable to join them in body, I did a quick search of the Web and found a live view from a camera mounted on the observatory at the summit. Pointed north, the camera showed the darkly hunched peaks of the northern Presidential Range beneath blue sky. Another click of the mouse gave me the current weather conditions. A near perfect July day: visibility 80 miles, wind at 35 miles per hour, temperature 42 degrees. Satisfied that my wife and son would experience the summit at its best, I then set out to discover, in their honor, what it might be possible to say about climbing, and not climbing. About remaining upright, and learning to fall.

Actors and stunt men learn to fall: as kids we watched them leap from moving trains and stage coaches. I have a dim memory of an eighth grade acting class in which I was taught to fall, but I can't remember the technique. Athletes learn to fall, and most people who have played sports have at some point had a coach tell them how to dive and roll, an art I never mastered. Devotees of the martial arts learn to fall, as do dancers and rock climbers. Mostly, though, we learn to do it badly.

My earliest memory: I'm standing alone at the top of the

stairs, looking down, scared. I call for my mother, but she doesn't come. I grip the banister and look down: I have never done this on my own before. It's the first conscious decision of my life. On some level I must know that by doing this I'm becoming something new: I am becoming an "I." The memory ends here: my hand gripping the rail above my head, one foot launched into space.

Forty years later, encroaching baldness has made it easier to see the scars I gained from that adventure. Still, I don't regret it. One has to start somewhere. Is not falling, as much as climbing, our birth right? In the Christian theology of the fall, we all suffer the fall from grace, the fall from our primordial connectedness with God. My little tumble down the stairs was my own expulsion from the Garden: ever after I have been falling forward and down into the scarred years of conscious life, falling into the knowledge of pain, grief, and loss.

We have all suffered, and will suffer, our own falls. The fall from youthful ideals, the waning of physical strength, the failure of a cherished hope, the loss of our near and dear, the fall into injury or sickness, and late or soon, the fall to our certain ends. We have no choice but to fall, and little say as to the time or the means.

Perhaps, however, we do have some say in the manner of our falling. That is, perhaps we have a say in matters of *style*. As kids we all played the game of leaping from a diving board or dock, and before hitting the water striking some outrageous or goofy pose: axe-murderer, Washington crossing the Delaware, rabid dog. Maybe it comes to no more than this. But I'd like to think that learning to fall is more than merely a matter of posing, more than an opportunity to play it for laughs. In fact I would have it that in the way of our falling we have the opportunity to express our essential humanity.

There's a well-known Zen parable about the man who was crossing a field when he saw a tiger charging at him. The man ran, but the tiger gained on him, chasing him toward the edge of a cliff. When he reached the edge, the man had no choice but to leap. He had one chance to save himself: a scrubby branch growing out of the side of the cliff about half way down. He grabbed the branch and hung on. Looking down, what did he see on the ground below? Another tiger.

Then the man saw that a few feet off to his left a small plant grew out of the cliff, and from it there hung one ripe strawberry. Letting go with one hand he found that he could stretch his arm out just far enough to pluck the berry with his fingertips and bring it to his lips.

How sweet it tasted!

I'm sure we've all found ourselves in this predicament.

I found myself in it summer before last, half way up the rock slide on the north peak of Mount Tripyramid. The north slide of Tripyramid is a mile of slick granite slabs and loose gravel partially grown over with scrubby spruce and birch on a pitch as steep as the roof of your house. I had done this hike as a boy, in canvas sneakers and long pants, but had not remembered how hard it was. Earlier that summer my weakening, wobbly legs had managed to get me up Chocorua with only a little trouble on the upper ledges. But here they had failed me. I had already fallen twice, bruising ribs, gashing knees, mashing one elbow to pulp. Standing there looking out over the valley, my legs shook and each breath brought pain. I had been in tight spots in the mountains before, but this was the closest I had ever felt to the entire wretched business of litters, rescue teams, and emergency vehicles. I looked out at the mountains because they were the only thing I could look at. The view down the slope at my feet was terrifying, the view up at the climb ahead intolerable.

Tigers either way.

In such a situation, one looks for blessings. As I stood there in pain looking neither up nor down but out across the valley to where granite peaks rose against a turbulent sky, I counted among my blessings the fact that it wasn't raining.

The steep rock slide, treacherous as it was now, would be deadly when wet. I had other blessings to count, as well. Three years into the course of an illness that kills most people in four or five, I belonged, statistically speaking, in a wheelchair, not on the side of a mountain. I was happy to be standing anywhere, and especially happy, all things considered, to be standing here, in my beloved White Mountains, looking out over miles of forested wilderness.

There was, however, that turbulent sky. Fact was, rain had been threatening all day. Those of you who have never stood in a high place and watched a rain storm move toward you across a valley have missed one of the things the words "awesome" and "majestic" were invented to describe. You're never quite sure you're seeing the rain itself: just a gray haze trailing below clouds drifting slow and steady as high sailed ships. Beautiful, yes, but in my present circumstances I felt something more than beauty. Seeing such a storm come at me now across that vast space I felt the astonishment of the sublime, which Edmund Burke defined in the eighteenth century as "not pleasure, but a sort of delightful horror, a sort of tranquillity tinged with terror." It was as though I had been privileged with a glimpse of my own death, and found it the most terrible and beautiful thing I had ever seen.

I suppose I could stop here and wrap all this up with a neat moral. I could give out the sort of advice you find in the magazines sold at the grocery store. You know what I mean. I've done my share of grocery shopping, and like all red-blooded American dads I reward myself by reading the women's magazines in the check-out line. Seems I can't get enough of "Three Weeks to Thinner Thighs," and "Ten Successful Men Tell What They Really Want in Bed." And I've always gotten my best parenting advice from *Working Mother* magazine. The articles in *Working Mother* follow a rigid formula: start with a catchy anecdote, then trot out an appropriately credentialed expert on whatever problem the anecdote was meant to illustrate—the whiny child, the fussy eater—then let the expert get down to the business of dishing out nuggets of advice set off in the text with bullet points. The formula is comforting and efficient. You know just what's coming, and if you're in a hurry you can skip the anecdote and credentials and get right to the bullet points.

I could do the same thing with the stories I've told so far. Surely the story of the tigers and my escapade on Mount Tripyramid yield nuggets of advice worthy of a bullet point or two:

- Don't wait for a tragedy to start appreciating the little things in life. We shouldn't have to be chased by tigers or leap off a cliff to savor the sweetness of a single strawberry.
- Stop and smell the honeysuckle. Or at least for goodness' sake stop and watch a rain storm the next time you see one.
- Count your blessings. Appreciate what you have instead of complaining about what you don't.

Now all of this is good advice. But I'm not writing this to give advice. I'm writing, I suppose, to say that life is not a problem to be solved. What do I mean by that? Surely life presents us with problems. When I have a toothache, I try to think rationally about its causes. I consider possible remedies, their costs and consequences. I might consult an expert, in this case a dentist, who is skilled in solving this particular sort of problem. And thus we get through much of life. As a culture we have accomplished a great deal by seeing life as a set of problems to be solved. We have invented new medicines, we have traveled to the moon, developed the computer on which I am writing this essay. We learned our method from the Greeks. From childhood on we are taught to be little Aristotles. We observe the world, we break down what we see into its component parts. We perceive problems and set about solving them, laying out our solutions in ordered sequences like the instructions for assembling a child's bicycle.

We have gotten so good at this method that we apply it to everything, and so we have magazine articles telling us the six ways to find a mate, the eight ways to bring greater joy into your life, the ten elements of a successful family, the twelve steps toward spiritual enlightenment. We choose to see life as a technical matter.

And here is where we go wrong. For at its deepest levels life is not a problem, but a mystery. The distinction, which I borrow from the philosopher Gabriel Marcel, is fundamental: problems are to be solved, true mysteries are not. Personally, I wish I could have learned this lesson more easily—without, perhaps, having to give up my tennis game. But each of us finds his or her own way to mystery. At one time or another, each of us confronts an experience so powerful, bewildering, joyous, or terrifying that all our efforts to see it as a "problem" are futile. Each of us is brought to the cliff's edge. At such moments we can either back away in bitterness or confusion, or leap forward into mystery. And what does mystery ask of us? Only that we be in its presence, that we fully, consciously, hand ourselves over. That is all, and that is everything. We can participate in mystery only by letting go of solutions. This letting go is the first lesson of falling, and the hardest.

I offer my stories not as illustrations of a problem, but as entrances into the mystery of falling. And now I'll offer not advice, not bullet points, but mystery points, set off in my text not with the familiar round dots but with question marks:

? If spiritual growth is what you seek, don't ask for more strawberries, ask for more tigers.

? The threat of the tigers, the leap from the cliff, are what give the strawberry its savor. They cannot be avoided, and the strawberry can't be enjoyed without them. No tigers, no sweetness.

? In falling we somehow gain what means most. In falling we are given back our lives even as we lose them.

My balance is not so good these days, and a short time before I began work on this essay last summer, I fell on the short path that leads through the woods from our driveway to the compost pile. I had just helped my six-year-old daughter into the car, and turned to start down the path, when I stumbled and went down hard. I lay stunned for a few moments, face numb, lip bleeding, chest bruised, my daughter Amelia standing over me asking, quite reasonably, what I was doing down there and whether I was all right. I wish I could have managed an answer such as "practicing my yoga" or "listening for hoofbeats." What I was doing was learning to fall. In the following days I did some thinking about the expression "watch your step," and even better, "mind your step." I thought about the Buddhist practice of walking meditation in which one becomes fully mindful of each step placed upon the earth. One of the blessings of my current stumbling condition is that I must practice this meditation continually, becoming mindful where I once was heedless. To walk upright upon the earth—what a blessing! When my wife and son left for their hike up Mount Washington and I set to work on this essay, I was also thinking about the expression "to fall on one's face," that perfect metaphor for those failures that cure us of complacency and pride.

The next day I learned that within minutes of my finishing a paragraph on these subjects and calling it quits for the afternoon, Kathryn found herself briefly airborne on Mount Washington. She and Aaron had made the summit, drunk in the gorgeous view I had peeped at via computer gimmickry, and then begun their descent down the treeless rock pile of the summit cone. Still well above treeline, on a steep slope approaching a precipice, her toe caught a rock and launched her up and out as though she intended a glider tour of the Great Gulf Wilderness. I can only imagine my son's thoughts as he watched his mother take flight, but surely my wife felt in those instants the pull toward twin possibilities for transcendence—upward toward some unearthly ascension and downward toward death—before crashing to the rocks, my son watching her bounce and roll toward the abyss, wondering if she would ever stop, Kathryn at last coming to rest, sorely convinced that her escape from earthly toil would not come so easily, in the meantime suffering the ordinary and decidedly untranscendent fate of three cracked ribs and a punctured lung.

What to make of all this? I'm a husband, but I'm also a writer, and even while making the necessary phone calls, dealing with the health insurance, and driving to the hospital, any writer worth his salt is on some level thinking, "this is good material." Writers, like bears, are willing to feed on almost anything.

Think again of falling as a figure of speech. We fall on our faces, we fall for a joke, we fall for someone, we fall in love. In each of these falls, what do we fall away from? We fall from ego, we fall from our carefully constructed identities, our reputations, our precious selves. We fall from ambition, we fall from grasping, we fall, at least temporarily, from reason. And what do we fall into? We fall into passion, into terror, into unreasoning joy. We fall into humility, into compassion, into emptiness, into oneness with forces larger than ourselves, into oneness with others whom we realize are likewise falling. We fall, at last, into the presence of the sacred, into godliness, into mystery, into our better, diviner natures.

After a few nights in the hospital and two difficult months my wife's ribs have mended. And I did make it to the top of Mount Tripyramid that day, despite the storm that splattered the rocks and sent us scurrying for rain gear. For I was not alone: my wife was there, and two of my brothers, and two young friends who hauled me, bloody and bowed, to the summit.

But this is not a story of triumph over adversity. The man chased by tigers does not win in the end, at least not Hollywood fashion. In Christian theology we fall so that we can rise again later. That's a good story, too, but not the one I'm telling today. I would rather, at least for now, find victory in the falling itself, in learning how to live fully, consciously in the presence of mystery. When we learn to fall we learn to accept the vulnerability that is our human endowment, the cost of walking upright on the earth.

In the northern part of our town there's a stream that comes down out of the mountains, and at one place that we call the Pothole it makes a pool of emerald clear water ten feet deep. Every summer from my boyhood until quite recently I would climb the rocks high above that pool and fling my body into the air. A summer was not complete without the thrill of that rushing descent, the slap of the water, the shock of its icy embrace. I have a photograph, taken two years ago, of what would prove to be my last such jump. In the foreground, seen from the back, my wife stands waist deep in water, shading her eyes with one hand, watching. She has never approved of this ritual, something most grown men leave behind with their teenage years, but there I am, half way down, pale against the dark rocks that I rush past. You can see my wet footprints on the rock over my head that I've just left. My eyes are focused downward on the water rushing toward my feet, and I am happy, terrified, alive.

We are all—all of us—falling. We are all, now, this moment, in the midst of that descent, fallen from heights that may now seem only a dimly remembered dream, falling toward a depth we can only imagine, glimpsed beneath the water's surface shimmer. And so let us pray that if we are falling from grace, dear God let us also fall *with* grace, *to* grace. If we are falling toward pain and weakness, let us also fall toward sweetness and strength. If we are falling toward death, let us also fall toward life.

2

GETTING UP IN THE MORNING (AND OTHER ESSENTIAL DUTIES)

Emperors don't get much airtime in American culture to day. And when we think of a stoic philosopher, we see a man in a toga with a bad haircut. To most of us stoicism means stuffing our feelings, shunning the pleasures of the flesh, and refusing to exercise our constitutional right to feel sorry for ourselves in public. So you may wonder what odd and possibly masochistic impulse has me wanting to write about Marcus Aurelius Antoninus, the Roman emperor and stoic.

Perhaps you'll forgive my eccentricities, seeing as everything I do these days I do with the urgency of a man whose days are numbered. Living with Lou Gehrig's disease, seeking both physical health and spiritual healing, I have learned to accept help from any quarter: I've consulted priests and shamans and psychics, bee keepers and body workers and aura balancers, naturopaths and homeopaths and neurologists, herbalists and acupuncturists and psychotherapists. I've even gone so far as to join a church and sing in the choir. Why not, then, seek help from a Roman emperor?

I don't mean to say that my diagnosis makes me special. Life, as I've said before, is a terminal condition. Those of us with terminal illnesses simply have been blessed—and I mean blessed—with having the facts of our own mortality held constantly before us. But we all bear the burdens of the flesh. And all of us at certain times in our lives, in the face of failure, loss, illness, and finally, our certain ends, find ourselves asking: why get up this morning? And, given what I'm facing, what work is there for me to do in this world that can possibly make a difference?

Lately I've come to feel quite strongly that answering these questions begins with acceptance. Not resignation, not passivity, but a profound and thorough acceptance of our place in the natural order. Not only must we accept our own deaths as a necessary part of that order, but we must come to see that it is our very mortality that calls us to act according to our highest nature. It is out of our acceptance of all that we are, including and especially that we are creatures that will one day die, that we are called to our highest human duties. Death, in other words, is good for us.

To explain how Marcus Aurelius Antoninus has helped me to understand these things, I'll have to go by way of the dump.

When I'm not teaching college in the Midwest, I live near my parents in a small town in New Hampshire where, as in many such towns, there are three real centers of civic life: the general store, the post office, and the dump. When I was spending summers there as a child about the only time I got to spend with my father was while we were working together on something, and so I have fond memories of our trips to the dump. The work was tedious and smelly, and I don't suppose we talked a whole lot, but it was good simply to be in my father's presence, admiring the manly assurance with which he hefted the barrels and bags into the back of the station wagon and drove us the few miles across town. In those days, the dump was a male realm, and for a boy like me—skinny, shy, awkward at sports—it was good to be initiated into its rituals: backing our load up to the heap, dropping the tailgate, then practicing my shot put form as I learned to balance a sack at my shoulder and one-handedly heave it up and out. A way of dancing, I suppose, and sacred in the way that all such ordinary dances are. Perhaps most satisfying was to see my father at ease in that setting, a man among men. My father worked long hours outside of the home; being quiet sorts, my folks didn't entertain much and, as the parents of five boys, were rarely invited to bring their children along to dinner parties. That's why, when the last empty barrel was thumped back in the station wagon, I was almost startled to hear my father hailed by another man, a friend or neighbor. Digging a hole with the toe of my boot, or pitching stones at seagulls, I would hide my joy at overhearing what to me was the rarest of things: easy, everyday, grownup male talk. It was as though the gods were speaking overhead and had allowed me to listen in. *Gods:* and my father was one of them!

Back then, the dump was really a dump. Once a week, from our home across town, we would see the air smudged with its burning. Nowadays, of course, it's not a dump but a "waste transfer facility," with its bins of colored glass and graded plastic, newspapers bundled with twine, and nonrecyclables hydraulically mashed in a dumpster to be hauled off on a truck to some prophylactic landfill far from the 100 square miles of swamp and granite ledge that is our town's portion of paradise. In fact, during my visit here last winter, there were engineers with clipboards overseeing the entombment, beneath layers of carefully graded gravel and plastic and clay, of that heap we so recklessly built and burned all the heedless days of my youth. Fortunately, some of the old ways die hard, and despite its new name everyone in town still calls the place "the dump." Even better, friends and neighbors still meet there to discuss the weather, exchange news, inquire after the sick, lobby their selectmen, arrange for carpentry, plumbing, and tree work, plot political strategy, and generally do the casual work of creating the sort of world fit for humans to live in.

The old ways also required that every dump have its dump man, that fellow whose job it was to keep an eye on things, but who spent most of his time, as everybody knew, huddled in his shack attending to the business of staying warm. Well, times being what they are, our town no longer has a dump man but a dump lady, and since she runs not a dump but a waste transfer facility, she spends less time keeping warm and more time keeping an eye on things. Also, times being what they are, our dump lady is a millionaire, having won the lottery a few years back. Sudden wealth has not lessened her zeal for her work, though. To the contrary: you go to the dump now anxiously, fearful that while emptying a few scraps of Sheetrock and old window screening into the compactor, Marge will descend upon you, all the scolding, bustling bulk of her, face asquint from the cigarette hanging in the corner of her mouth, directing you firmly to the building materials Dumpster, and perhaps even suggesting an extra fee for disposing of that suspicious looking pile of paint cans in the back of your pickup truck. A former factory worker who prefers the dump because the town pays health insurance, Marge is the best there is: aggressive, exacting, a professional.

It is another New Hampshire tradition that you go to the dump not simply to throw out your trash but to look for things that might be useful. There's a saying that you know you're really from New Hampshire if you leave the dump with more than you came with. Marge helps out here, sorting out useful items and setting them aside in an area she calls The Swap Shop. When my wife and I were building and furnishing our house here, Marge began setting aside things she thought we might like, and her swap shop provided us with several windows, a screen door, a fine old rocking chair for the porch, a set of glassware, waffle iron, blender, toaster oven, children's books, clothing, and an old feather bed. In New Hampshire, where thrift is a household god, there is no shame attached to such scavenging. Most people here have someplace at home where they tuck away things that might be useful at some future date. The poet Donald Hall has suggested that instead of "Live Free or Die" New Hampshire license plates should read "It Might Come In Handy."

The best place to keep all those things that might come in handy is, of course, the barn. Our barn actually serves as my wife's sculpture studio, and one day last summer I saw that Kathryn had put a row of books on a shelf amidst her sculptor's tools. These books, salvaged from Marge's swap shop, were not texts to be read but sculptural materials to be hacked, drilled, sawed, lacquered, slathered in plaster and cast in bronze. (This is a woman who has married a writer and professor of English literature. While fifty yards away I'm in my cabin in the woods *writing* books, she's in her studio inflicting various tortures upon them, and in this regard you could say we have the perfect marriage.) As chance would have it, on that day I rescued from her shelf one small leatherbound volume, a 1929 edition, printed in Great Britain, of *The Meditations of the Emperor Marcus Aurelius Antoninus*, a book I had heard much about but never read.

I took an immediate liking to Aurelius. He slept on a bare board, ate little, prayed to his gods, and commanded an empire. He thought continually of his own death, and when I read his words I knew I had met a soul worth reckoning with:

> Let it make no difference to thee whether thou art cold or warm, if thou art doing thy duty; and whether thou art drowsy or satisfied with sleep; and whether ill-spoken or praised; and whether dying or doing something else. For it is one of the acts of life, this act

by which we die: it is sufficient then in this act also to
do well what we have in hand.

Whether dying *or doing something else*. The casualness of
that phrase! I imagine Aurelius getting off of his board in the
morning and making his to-do list for the day:

1. Breakfast with Faustina
2. Address the Senate on the need to defend the northern frontier
3. Prune rose bushes, sacrifice goat.
4. Die?
5. If not, lead army against the barbarians.

Apparently, Aurelius wrote his meditations as notes to
himself, for his own benefit. He reveres the natural order,
writing that "all things are implicated with one another, and
the bond is holy." For him, to be connected to all things and
all people is to be humbled, for "Asia, Europe are corners of
the universe: all the sea a drop in the universe; Athos a little
clod of the universe: all the present time a point in eternity."

Because all things are connected, good and bad are connected, too, and deserve equally our reverence:

> All things are little, changeable, perishable. All things
> come from god, from that universal ruling power ...
> And accordingly the lion's gaping jaws, and that which
> is poisonous, and every harmful thing, as a thorn, as
> mud, are after-products of the grand and beautiful. Do
> not then imagine that they are of another kind from
> that which thou venerate, but form a just opinion of
> them all.

Our challenge, then, is to accept all that befalls us as belonging to the natural order, to see nothing that happens to
us as foreign:

> Nothing can happen to any man which is not a human accident, nor to an ox which is not according to the nature of an ox, nor to a vine which is not according to the nature of a vine, nor to a stone which is not proper to a stone. If then there happens to each thing both what is usual and natural, why shouldst thou complain? For the common nature brings nothing which may not be borne by thee.

Among life's other accidents, we must accept death:

> Do not despise death, but be well content with it, since this too is one of those things which nature wills .... As thou waitest for the time when the child shall fall out of thy wife's womb, so be ready for the time when thy soul shall fall out of this envelope.

To accept death is to live with a profound sense of freedom. The freedom, first, from attachment to the things of this life that don't really matter: fame, material possessions, and even, finally, our own bodies. Acceptance brings the freedom to live fully in the present. The freedom, finally, to act according to our highest nature:

> Everywhere and at all times it is in thy power piously to acquiesce in thy present condition, and to behave justly to those about thee.

Only when we accept our present condition can we set aside fear and discover the love and compassion that are our highest human endowments. And out of our compassion we deal justly with those about us. Not just on our good days, not just when it's convenient, but *everywhere and at all times* we are free to act according to that which is highest in us. And in such action we find peace.

But it is with acceptance that we must begin.

To see what that might look like, let's go back to the dump.

The reason our dump is now a waste transfer facility and not a dump is that a hundred yards downhill from the dump is a swamp dammed up by beavers to make a shallow, reedy pond, and out of that pond in the early summer the snapping turtles crawl up on land looking for a place to lay their eggs. One day I went to the dump with my own son, Aaron, who was then six years old. We arrived to see a turtle making its nest in a pile of sand that had been bulldozed to the dump's edge. She had laid her eggs in a pit about a foot deep and two feet across, but by the time we got there, Marge had already removed the eggs from the nest to save them from the raccoons, planning to incubate them at home and return the hatchlings to the swamp. If the turtle knew that the eggs were gone, she seemed unconcerned, and what my son and I watched was a snapping turtle with a shell the size of a hubcap trying to crawl out of a sandy hole.

No matter how many times you've heard the story of the tortoise and the hare, you have never really understood it until you've watched a turtle get where it needs to go. She had a bad time of it. The sand was loose, and the sides of the pit kept crumbling beneath her, tumbling her back to the bottom. Each time she fell, she resumed her climb without pause, stubby legs churning at the same slow, relentless pace, webbed claws shoveling sand behind her, her prehistoric head with its fabled jaw thrust forward, implacable as time itself. Pathetically, she made no progress, and after a while we turned to the business of dumping trash and sorting bottles, as I explained to my son that Marge or somebody would eventually help her out.

But that didn't happen. By the time Aaron and I had finished our chores and turned to look again, the turtle was gone. No one had helped her. Though we had not been attending to her business, *she* clearly had, and now she was down in the swamp again, getting on with whatever else needed doing that day.

I have seen other turtles. Out driving in early summer you'll encounter them on the roads where the road dips to cross a stream. I once stopped my car in the middle of a bridge to let one cross. It must have climbed out of the stream some fifteen feet below, and I got out of my car to watch it haul itself across the asphalt until it reached the bridge's edge, and then, not knowing it was on a bridge, tip over the edge to plunge back down into the stream from which it had come. Though I don't know how the turtle felt about this, I felt awful. But while I was busy entertaining my frustration at the wasted effort, while I was busy making the turtle's fall an emblem for all the botched beginnings and abrupt endings of my days, the turtle was busy swimming to the shore and haul-ing itself out to begin the long climb up the bank again. As if to say to me, where I stood swaddled in my mooning and moaning self, as if to say, "See? See how I dance? See how it's done?"

I was in the kitchen one day with my daughter Amelia, who is six years old. My children know that my hands give me trouble now with little things—all the zippers and clasps and buckles and screws with which we like to think we hold our world together—and Amelia must have remarked on this, and then our conversation went this way:

"My hands don't work very well, but I can still hug you."

"And what if your arms don't work?" she asked.

"Then you'll have to hug *me*," I said. "As long as you hug me, I'll be okay."

Now, my daughter has a lawyer's precision and a nose for cheap sentiment.

"Well, *Papa*," she said, "if I don't hug you, you can still *survive*."

There's nothing to say to this, of course. She knows what the turtle knows, and she's right. I can survive. And, being human, I know more: not only that I can survive, but that I am blessed. Each day that I can get out of bed in the morning, I am blessed. Each day that any of us can move our limbs to do the world's work, we are blessed. And if limbs wither, and speech fails, we are still blessed. So long as this heart beats, I am blessed, for it is our human work, it is our human duty, finally, to rise each day in the face of loss, to rise in the face of grief, of debility, of pain, to move as the turtle moves, her empty nest behind her, her labor come to nothing, up out of the pit and toward the next season's doing.

There's a Native American story about how the turtle got the cracks in its shell. One day the turtle walking through the forest met a flock of birds all noisy and excited about going south. The turtle was curious, and asked if they could take her with them. Two of the birds held a stick between them with their feet, and the turtle clamped onto it with her powerful jaws, and in that way they lifted the turtle up and away over the forest. The turtle was dazzled by the view from up there, and wanted the birds to explain it all to her. She waggled her arms and legs to get their attention, but the birds took no notice and went on speaking over her head of their own affairs. Then the turtle grunted and groaned with the same results. When at last she could stand it no longer, the turtle opened her mouth to ask the birds what all these things were that she was seeing. That, of course, was a mistake, for now she found the forest rushing up to meet her. She pulled in her head, her arms, and legs, and whap, struck the ground flat on her back. And that's how the turtle's shell got cracked. But the turtle was lucky, for she landed near a pond. She managed to drag her bruised and aching body into the cool water, and then to burrow into the oozy, healing mud at the bottom, and there sleep till spring. To this day the turtle bears those cracks upon its shell to remind it that it's not a bird. And we bear our bodies, our fabulous and failing bodies, to remind us that we're humans and not angels.

No fancy moral here. Simple truths are hardest. I get out of bed every morning to attend to the business of being human, whether that business happens to be dying or doing something else. I get out of bed in the morning to do what good remains within my power to do.

And each day, in a small New Hampshire town, Marge, a millionaire, rises early to get to the dump, to see that all our leavings are well left, to sort the useful from the useless, and to keep from the ground all that might seep to the swamp below, so that beavers will still do their work, and the water rise, and the turtles thrive there and in the early summers crawl on the land to make their nests, some of them finding their way to the dump, where in years to come other fathers and other sons, doing their work together, will see them, and know this way of dancing.

3

IN PRAISE OF THE IMPERFECT LIFE

All winter the beech trees hold a few leaves, reminding us of what we've lost. Even into April, as buds fatten, the old leaves hang on, pale scraps rasping in wind. From a passing car you see them, scattered through the woods like litter caught in branches. Then one day they're gone. The new leaves have split their shells and pushed the old ones off. Good riddance, we might well say. Spring has been long in coming, and we're ready to get on with it. For a few weeks as the trees unfold their wrinkled leaves we're staggered by good fortune; we wander out through fields, snuffling the loamy scent of earth warmed more deeply by the hour. We tilt our faces sunward, celebrating with e.e. cummings "the leaping greenly spirits of trees / and a blue true dream of sky." We squish mud between our toes. We press our faces into flowers. After five months of iron earth and wind-driven snow and sleet, we have earned our spring revel.

Yet some part of me holds back. To balance e.e. cummings, I need Robert Frost's warning that these trees "have it in their pent-up buds / To darken nature and be summer woods." Spring *is* a darkening. The shade thickens about my house;

my view of the Ossipee Mountains vanishes behind the fringe of trees at the far edge of the field. The vernal pools in the woods below our field will soon be gone, as Frost observes, "not out by any brook or river, / But up by roots to bring dark foliage on." Spring enlivens us, yet from our human vantage not all resurrections are equally welcome. Our allergies awaken with the flowers, pine pollen sifts a yellow film over the furniture. Our neighborhood bear, newly tumbled from his den and hungry as—well, a bear—rouses the household at 3 a.m., trashing the bird feeder and terrorizing the dog. And then, in case we still thought all was perfect in paradise, the insects arrive.

If you don't live in the north woods, you won't understand what I mean by this. Vacationers who come for a week in August have little idea that the year-round folks have just survived plagues rivaling those visited on Pharaoh's Egypt. From early May to late July, the in-crowd's exoskeletal. Ticks make an early go of it: climbing to the tips of grass blades, they will hitch a ride on any passing mammal but seem to prefer me. After a half hour's walk in the field I find a dozen crawling up my legs. They hide in clothes, in sheets. I wake to the sensation of one plodding up my back, seeking a place to burrow and bloat.

Luckily, we have black flies to take our minds off the ticks. Black flies look like mouse droppings with wings. Outdoors in late May, each of us travels with his or her own swarm. Around town you see gardeners shrouded with olive drab bug-net helmets, as though ready to handle plutonium. Black flies don't sting, they bite, leaving us pocked with scabs that we tear off when scratching. The flies crawl up sleeves and noses, burrow into ears. If New Hampshire people are tight lipped, perhaps it's that black flies have taught us the cost of opening our mouths.

All nature clamors for our blood, and who can blame it? Bugs seek nothing we don't seek for ourselves: to eat before being eaten, to be fruitful and multiply. But what designing genius fashioned the mosquito? Who decided that it needed seven mouth parts—no more, no less—to grip and drill and pump and suck? And who developed the tag team format whereby, just as the mosquitoes tire in July, the deer flies arrive to burrow through our sun-warmed hair and chew our scalps?

There are advantages, I suppose, to living in a country under siege. For one thing, the bugs, along with the winters, keep the human population in check. Or, counting your blessings, you could say that only during bug season does your skin feel fully alive. And if, like me, you're a philosophical sort, you might welcome the bugs as a spiritual challenge, and ask what they can tell us about the place of suffering and imperfection in our lives.

All right, I admit it. I suppose it *is* perverse of me to go outdoors on a breezy, sunny spring morning, and walk past wildflowers nodding in the meadow down to my quiet cabin in the woods, all so that I can shut myself up and think about suffering. Well, it's tough work, but somebody's got to do it. And perhaps my life circumstances have pushed me, more insistently than most, to consider how a flawed life can still be a full one, how broken dreams can bring us more fully awake.

Traditional religion teaches us to accept our afflictions as belonging to a larger scheme beyond mortal grasp. We're to trust the one or ones in charge. As I heard one unhappy young woman say recently, "I guess God's got his rhymes and reasons." It was late on a Friday afternoon, in the employees' lounge of a school for developmentally disabled children, and at the end of a long week a child in this woman's care had been hospitalized for seizures. It would indeed be comforting to think that the suffering of these children, with their scrambled circuits and skewed limbs, belonged to some larger dispensation of justice and mercy. But this woman did not feel comforted. Laying her head on her arms, she announced her intention to cash her paycheck, go home, and drink herself numb.

But maybe we're asking the wrong thing of God. Rhyme and reason, after all, are human values, not divine ones. Wanting human suffering to fit some divine plan is like wanting to fly an airplane above tornado wreckage and see that it spells out song lyrics or a cure for acne. At some point in life, in the face of illness, violence, accident, or injustice, each of us confronts the possibility that rhyme and reason may not be on God's agenda. This, of course, leads many people to dispense with God and religion altogether. In workshops I've led, when people explain their reasons for turning away from religion, most often I've heard them cite some instance of suffering, either global or personal: religion hasn't ended war; it doesn't explain why a boy's sister had to die of leukemia. I'm not sure how to answer such charges except to suggest that perhaps we shouldn't turn to religion for solutions and explanations of this sort. The first of Buddhism's Four Noble Truths is the one that our experience most easily confirms: that to be human is to suffer. God, the power that creates and sustains the universe in each moment and has given us our very lives, doesn't owe us *reasons*.

In the biblical tradition, no one learns this lesson more powerfully than Job. Job, you'll recall, is that cosmic schlimazel who has the misfortune of being around when God, on a sort of dare from Satan, decides to test a good man's faith. Though Job is an upright and pious man, his children are killed, his worldly goods destroyed. Job responds by tearing his clothes, shaving his head, and falling to the ground in worship, saying, "Naked I came from my mother's womb, and naked shall I return there; the Lord gave, and the Lord has taken away; blessed be the name of the Lord." But this doesn't satisfy Satan, who argues that Job is merely bargaining for his life. To test him further, God allows Job to be covered "from the sole of his foot to the crown of his head in loathsome sores." Job then retires to sit in the ashes, scraping his sores with a piece of broken pottery, and cursing the day he was born.

At this point Job's wife, wishing an end to her husband's suffering, urges Job to "curse God, and die."

And here Job makes the most extraordinary answer: "Shall we receive good at the hand of God, and not receive the bad?"

In these words I find a challenge that shakes me to the core. For those who dismiss traditional religion as offering a simplified and sentimental version of reality, Job offers a darker, more complex vision than those we may remember being taught in Sunday school. For those who think reason has the final say in human affairs, Job reminds us how little reason avails us when we try to understand all that befalls us. For those who are religious yet want to think of God only as the God of goodness and love, for those for whom prayer is always a turning toward the light, for those of us who seek in spiritual experience nothing but sweetness and harmony, Job offers a severer, more inclusive view. "Shall we receive good at the hand of God, and not receive the bad?" Job now knows that God is the God of good *and* of evil, light *and* darkness, sweet *and* bitter, harmony *and* discord. Hindus embody this truth in the god Shiva, who both creates and destroys. The Koranic phrase, *La'illaha il'Allahu*, teaches there is nothing that is not from God, that everything, birth and death, joy and suffering, the green spurt of youth and the slow decay of age, bread and excrement, our sweetest singing and our cries of agony, all of it is from God.

When God finally does speak to Job, out of the whirlwind, he doesn't come to explain himself. Among the most powerful rhetorical passages in all literature, God's tongue-lashing of Job boils down to saying: "I'm God, and you're not." Before God makes his appearance, Job has eloquently argued his innocence before his friends, who assume that Job's troubles must be punishment for some wrongdoing. And even though Job is right—he really is innocent—once God arrives on the scene, Job sees that his arguments are worthless. In the presence of the creator of the universe, he can do nothing but fall silent and "repent in dust and ashes," surrendering all he thought most precious: his intelligence, his reputation, his righteousness, his rhymes and his reasons, his very self. In that wordless place, beyond all niggling over right and wrong, Job's surrender moves us toward a wholeness and connectedness in which *all* things, good and evil, are divine, all part of the sacred dance of creation. And in confronting Job's vision, in facing every day the failure of my own flesh, in facing every day the reality of suffering all around me, I have found my life's greatest spiritual challenge.

The title of this essay was inspired by a poem by Wallace Stevens. "The Poems of Our Climate" begins with the lines: "Clear water in a brilliant bowl / pink and white carnations." It's a conventional poetic image of beauty and perfection: a bowl of flowers, pure, simple, and, well, *dull*. The poem goes on to argue that even if one could achieve such purity and simplicity, "one would want more, one would need more," for "there would still remain the never-resting mind" calling us back from the cold purity of perfection to the hot, bitter delight of human imperfection. The poem's climactic line announces the truth at the heart of this book: "The imperfect is our paradise."

There are two ways to seek God, Stevens' poem reminds me. The first way fixes on images of beauty and perfection, shunning all that is evil and ugly. This was Plato's way. When Plato banished the poets from his ideal Republic, he did so to protect the impressionable young from depictions of ugliness and evil. Plato insisted that enlightenment could be attained only by training the mind on the good. But then there is the other way, the dark way, the path of imperfection and suffering. This is the way of Dante, who, following Jesus' example, knew that to reach Paradise he had to travel through the Inferno. Dante's way is also the way of Job, and the way expressed by the Sufi poet Jalal al-Din Rumi when he writes:

> Be a full bucket,
> drawn up the dark way of a well,
> then lifted out,
> into the light.

I have become, perhaps by force of necessity, a seeker of the second kind, a seeker of the dark way of the well, traveling upward toward the light, but knowing that in the end some force larger than me must lift me out.

I say that I'm now a seeker of this second kind, but it wasn't always so. Once I was a seeker of the first kind, on the path of beauty and perfection. In my spiritual questing through my teens and twenties, I sought transcendence, enlightenment, bliss. I learned meditation, retreated alone into the wilderness, and experimented with drugs, waiting for the transforming vision, for the voices of angels robed in fire. I sought God in the extraordinary, in things not of this world.

The summer after I finished college I took a bus to California, and after various adventures sublime and sordid, I hitchhiked to a religious commune that I knew of, in the basin and range country of eastern Nevada, a land of sagebrush and dust, jackrabbits and coyotes and rattlesnakes and antelope, a few cattle and fewer people. At the base of the Snake Range, this commune was no hippie hangout, no faddish Age of Aquarius retreat but a community founded in the 1930's by a Methodist minister's son who had spent years studying yoga with an Indian spiritual master. I spent a week at the commune, doing farm chores: I learned to pick apricots, to make a garden fence that deer couldn't jump over. I learned that before you chop a chicken's head off, you should swing the chicken by the feet to calm it down. But for much of my time there I meditated and studied, did breath work and kundalini yoga, seeking the sort of mystical, transforming experience that to me constituted the one true glamour of the spiritual life.

At the end of the week I went up into the mountains, for there above the farm the peaks of the Snake Range rose to 13,000 feet. Now it so happens that on the shoulder of the highest peak there lives a grove of bristle-cone pine trees, some of them over 5,000 years old, the oldest living things on earth. Having been a tree-worshiper from a young age, I saw a journey to these trees as a fitting end to my pilgrimage. So I got a ride up the narrow road that takes you to about 9,000 feet and then hiked in several miles until I came upon them. Perhaps you have seen them in photographs: gnarled trees, seeming almost lifeless, the bark blasted from their gray weathered trunks except for one thin lifeline that snakes up to sustain the green bottle-brush needles. These grotesque forms grow where nothing else survives; in a high place of wind and snow and stone they push up through glacial rubble with their delicate offering of green. I walked among them, in silence, while sheer walls of stone rose above me a thousand feet to jagged peaks, their crevices veined with ice. Though this was July, snowfields slumped at the shadowed base of the cliffs. Turning my back to the cliffs, I could look out across thirty miles of sagebrush valley to where the next range of peaks glittered in sunlight. If ever there was a place for transcendence, I told myself, this was it. On the tortured trunk of a tree several thousand years old, I found one sticky, golden drop of bristle-cone sap, which I plucked off and solemnly placed on my tongue, wishing for long life. And then I prepared to meditate. Settling down with my back against the ancient tree's trunk, my legs crossed, my spine erect, the sun warm on my face, a gentle breeze lifting the hair on my forearms, I closed my eyes, ready for my vision.

I waited. I waited some more. I quieted my thoughts, stilled my breath.

It began as an itch, a small one, low down on my back, something that with discipline I could ignore. I bore down, counted my breath, focused on my crown chakra. The itch had become a tickle, and moved higher on my back, disturbing my focus. I held on, projecting a cone of white light from my crown to the heavens, seeking contact. The tickle rose between my shoulder blades, becoming a torment, and I could bear it no longer: I writhed and scratched, trying to hang on to my perfect moment.

What was this thing? Was *this* the stirring of the kundalini energy, rising up through my chakras, heralding my enlightenment?

No. It was an ant. An ant had crawled up inside my shirt, on business known only to itself. It was stubborn and elusive, and after more violent contortions, my meditation spoiled, I removed my shirt, shook out the ant, and spent the rest of the afternoon rambling over the rocks before hiking down to the road.

I had come for a miracle. What I got was an ant.

Only now, years later, have I come to understand that the ant *was* the miracle.

More than in those ancient trees, more than in the mountains, more than in the vast space stretching out before me, the true nature of God was revealed to me in the humble climbing of an ant, after an intriguing smell, perhaps, or the pleasing salty taste of skin. It was the ant that returned me to the world, that called me to another way of worship, the way of all things ordinary and small, the way of all that is imperfect, the way of stubbornness and error, the way of all that is transitory and comes to grief. The ant was my messenger, calling me back to a world that in truth I had never left. As T.S. Eliot writes:

> We shall not cease from exploration
> And the end of all our exploring

Will be to arrive where we started
And know the place for the first time.

And so I have returned to become a seeker of the second kind, a seeker of the dark way. I've grown suspicious of perfection, seeking not a perfect life but a full one. We have all had our magic moments, when we enter that forest clearing where dragonflies dance and sunlight descends as a kind of grace. But we know such bright moments only because of the darkness that surrounds them. The clearing needs the forest, and I've learned to be thankful for its shadows.

The other day, my wife, my children, and I watched toads breeding at Bearcamp Pond. Their loud trilling drew us to the sheltered lagoon where toads slid and tumbled over one another in the shallows. Our eyes were drawn to one mating pair, the smaller male clinging to the larger female's back, out in deeper water, now sinking, now rising to the surface, now resting, now stroking their rear legs together, a languorous and lovely dance. Not for some time did we see, with a slight shift of focus, the snapping turtle just below—an old giant, half boulder, half jaw, big as a hassock—waiting in the depths to devour them. Who's to say where God lies?

We have all heard poems, songs, and prayers that exhort us to see God in a blade of grass, a drop of dew, a child's eyes, or the petals of a flower. Now when I hear such things I say that's too *easy*. Our greater challenge is to see God not only in the eyes of the suffering child but in the suffering itself. To thank God for the sunset pink clouds over Red Hill—but also for the mosquitoes I must fan from my face while watching the clouds. To thank God for broken bones and broken hearts, for everything that opens us to the mystery of our humanness. The challenge is to stand at the sink with your hands in the dishwater, fuming over a quarrel with your spouse, children at your back clamoring for attention, the radio blatting the bad news from Bosnia, and to say "God is here, now, in this room, here in this dishwater, in this dirty spoon." Don't talk to me about flowers and sunshine and waterfalls: this is the ground, here, now, in all that is ordinary and imperfect, this is the ground in which life sows the seeds of our fulfillment.

The imperfect is our paradise.

Let us pray, then, that we do not shun the struggle. May we attend with mindfulness, generosity, and compassion to all that is broken in our lives. May we live fully in each flawed and too human moment, and thereby gain the victory.

4

UNFINISHED HOUSES

Even as a child I shared my mother's fascination with houses. Driving around town on errands or taking me and my brothers to the beach, she would comment on old houses we drove past. Sometimes she and I would go out just to look at some house that had recently been put up for sale. I remember once turning up a dirt drive into a yard gone to foot-high grass and weeds. It was summer, with the smell of summer dust and heat, katydids fluttering up at each step, and behind the house, crickets chorusing in a neglected field that was filling with juniper and birch. We worked our way around the old white clapboard farmhouse, peering through windows, our shoes crunching the stubbled remains of flower beds. Hands cupped against my forehead, nose to the glass, I gazed through the glare into a succession of empty rooms, sensing in those worn floorboards, skewed doorframes, and faded floral wallpapers the possibilities for another life from the one I knew.

My mother had no intention of buying. We were already settled into an old white clapboard farmhouse of our own. I say we were settled, but perhaps this was not entirely so. Our house, like most in these parts, was a work in progress. Already my parents had reshingled the back wall, installed a large kitchen window to give us a view of the Ossipee mountains, reclaimed an ancient fireplace hidden behind wallboard, torn down the two-hole privy leaning off the back of the ell and replaced it with a set of steps, and made enough plans for future changes to keep them busy for years. Ralph Waldo Emerson once wrote that "people wish to be settled; only so far as they are unsettled is there any hope for them." I suppose that with her restless interest in other houses, her continued improvement of our own, her ceaseless imagining of other possibilities for herself and her family, there was, and still is, hope for my mother. And I want to consider what hope there might be for all of us who in some way or other remain unsettled.

I am writing this in January, and if ever there was a time of year to be settled, this is it. Here in New England preparing for winter is a year-round occupation, and by now we've long ago gotten the wood in, staked the driveway for the plow, and watched the first snows bury our summer's work in garden, yard, and field. Here in winter's deep, dark time, a season that finds us denned, burrowed, and hunkered through long nights and brief days, it may seem foolish to search for some virtue in being unsettled in our houses. But let me do my best, in the spirit of Emerson when he writes "I unsettle all things."

My mother's interest in houses is part of a larger history. When my parents came up from Massachusetts looking for a country house, they were part of a wave of such people that lasted through the 1950s and '60s. Our town's population had reached a low of around 600 people, lower than it had been since soon after the town's founding in the late 1700s. My parents' cohort bought and renovated old houses all over town, employing a growing number of younger tradesmen and craftsmen who in turn bought and built houses of their own and now with their families have doubled the town's year-round population and made Sandwich the happy small place it is today. So it's no wonder that we're interested in houses, and that everyone I know is happy to talk at length about them. Ours is not the bland talk of real estate prices and interest rates that you hear in suburban communities. In my town you're expected to know your girts from your beams, your headers from your ledgers, your rafters from your collar ties. At church suppers, at our children's birthday parties, on the sidelines at soccer practice, or during intermission at the Christmas concert, we talk stud walls and stress-skin panels and Typar and hurricane bracing; we talk vapor barriers and blueboard and polyisocyanurate insulation; we talk shallow wells and drilled wells, septic tanks and leaching fields. You have never witnessed passion until you've heard your neighbors discourse on the virtues of full-dimension lumber or low-e glass. The words themselves are charged, erotic, tasted in the mouth like delicacies: *shiplap, splined boards, tongue and groove.*

Maybe it's because we so enjoy talking about our houses that we never finish them. After all, if we finished them, what would we have to talk about? So we leave drywall unpainted, closets without doors, windows without trim. We live for years with plywood subfloors over which someday we fully intend to install the wide-board oak of our dreams. Fact is, almost no one I know here lives in an entirely finished house, and those few who do are embarrassed to admit it. And whether our houses are finished or not, most of us have a drawer somewhere with sketches of various rooms and outbuildings yet to be constructed. I know that in some places people live differently. I know there are places, lying south of Concord, I suppose, where people move into finished houses, where everything is spic and span, the windows washed and the hinges oiled and even the clock on the stove set to the right time. But this is the country, and we live differently.

This essay was inspired by a friend of mine, recently returned to town after a year away, who planned on renting a house for the winter. The house was unfinished, with exposed insulation in the walls. No matter: my friend, the single mother of a ten-year-old boy, whose family has been in this town for 150 years, said that she would "just throw up some Sheetrock." What struck me was not only her resilience and good spirit in the face of challenge, but that she could assume, correctly, that I would think "throwing up some Sheetrock" to make a house livable for the winter not at all an unusual thing to do. This is a place where respectable people staple plastic over their windows, stack hay bales against their foundations. If our town were a country, its national flag would be the blue tarp. Thrown over leaky roofs, old cars, and unfinished outbuildings, it's a fitting symbol of a nation dedicated to the provisional and the temporary. Its cheerful presence outside our houses proclaims the frugality and craftiness with which we cheat time and our own limitations.

What else keeps us from finishing our houses? Reasons are not hard to find: we lack the money, or choose to spend it otherwise; those of us who insist on doing the work ourselves are too busy with other chores, including the eternal chore of making a living. In most cases we simply get used to things as they are, and the pain of unfinished tasks diminishes to a dull and manageable ache. Still, a certain shame remains, and we show visitors the unfinished features of our houses with a look of hangdog guilt at our own inefficiency and sloth. This guilt, however, barely conceals a deeper pride. Those of us who are non-natives have come here, we know, for therapy, as part of a lifelong project of getting in touch with our "inner Yankee." A degree of make-do shabbiness is required to show we are making progress. Yankees, whether by birth or adoption, have always found ways to let their neighbors know the extent of their thrift and stoicism, and native and newcomer alike find a too-finished house as out of place as a mink coat worn to the post office.

But when we push even deeper we discover yet another level of feeling: not guilt, not pride, but despair. For on our bad days, in our dark moments, we see in our unfinished houses the surest sign of calamity. That unpainted drywall, that missing piece of trim remind us that the world is too much with us, that we have lost our grip, that life hurls more at us than we can handle. At such times we find ourselves aboard time's driverless train, rushing toward doom. For we know, don't we, that we will never get it all done, that we are never good enough, and that surely it will all get away from us, that our fields will fill with brush, our stone walls topple, our houses collapse and sink into the earth to become more of the cellar holes scattered through these woods and hills like so many monuments to failure.

Such dark days have their flip side, of course, when in manic rebound we indulge our fantasies: for we also know, don't we, that someday when our kids are grown, when our ex-husbands finally pony up with child support, when we sell that screenplay, when we get that new job selling condo time-shares, when we have *really* figured out the World Wide Web, when we finally learn to balance our checkbooks, when all our ships come sailing in, all our cows are cashed, when maple trees grow money, when at last our lives take that stunning upswing and we ascend into the glittering hoo-hah of a destiny we knew all along was ours, then, *then* we'll put cedar shingles on that wall that has been wrapped in Typar since our children were born, *then* we will drill a deep well so that our teenage daughters can take endless hot showers and we can water our tomatoes until they grow fat, *then* we will install a radiant floor heating system so that we can walk cozily barefoot in February, *then* we will add on that master bedroom suite with the indoor Jacuzzi and the outdoor hot tub, *then* we'll build that cupola with the hammock hanging in it from which we can gaze at stars. And then will all the scattered pieces of ourselves be gathered up, all that has been lost returned to us, all our wounds healed, all our griefs assuaged, and all our days will pass in happiness, our nights in bliss.

But that hasn't happened yet, has it? Fact is, most of us make do with our duct tape and blue tarps, our patched and cobbled houses giving physical form to all that remains unfinished and imperfect in our own cramped and needful selves. Don't get me wrong: I love my house. Sitting with a cup of coffee at the table, basking in the low January sun that fills our house with light while outside spindrift whips over the fields, I am the luckiest man on God's frozen earth. Still, most of us most of the time, and all of us some of the time, live in houses that remind us of the many ways in which life has turned out to be *not quite what we had in mind.*

My unsettling suggestion is that perhaps this is a good thing.

Our houses, like our lives, will never be finished, never be settled. The only thing that will settle the affairs of this life is death itself. To be too settled in this life is, in Emerson's sense, to die while still living, to live a sort of death-in-life. Only so far as we are unsettled is there any hope for us. Let us remain unsettled, therefore, in order that we may truly live.

But to follow this line of inquiry further, I need to tell you now about Orrin Tilton, and how he lived and died. That old clapboard farmhouse we lived in when I was a child was on Tilton Hill Road, and when we moved there the last Tilton still living on the road was our next door neighbor. When I first knew him, Orrin Tilton was a man in his 50s, living with his disabled father in a house that hadn't seen paint in decades and was heated by the monstrous Glenwood cookstove in a kitchen lit by a single bare bulb. Orrin's father, I remember, used to sit in a chair in the kitchen, or in the yard when it was warm, and try to sell us wood scraps from a bucket he kept at his feet.

Orrin, like many New Hampshire folk who had seen an

entire agricultural world vanish around them, made his living as a carpenter and handyman, occasionally firing up his old tractor to hay the field he still owned across from our house. He was not given to idle talk; about the most flamboyant thing he ever did was on one Fourth of July, when he fired off his antique brass cannon using the supply of black powder that he stored under his bed. But in those first years he helped us flatlanders get settled in, steering my father patiently over the shoals of cranky plumbing, shallow wells and rotting sills. He refinished our pine floors and put a new roof on our barn, and sometimes my mother had him over for a spaghetti supper. I remember him most clearly as he sat at our table, a wiry man with strongly muscled arms, thin, close-cropped gray hair, ears that stood well out from his head, gray eyes that swam behind thick lenses, and a drop of spaghetti sauce on his chin.

Years later, when as a teenager I lay in bed late at night memorizing Robert Frost's poem "An Old Man's Winter Night," it was Orrin Tilton I imagined clomping through his empty house, going about the humble and ordinary business of putting himself and all the countryside he cared for to bed, while outside, ominously, "all out of doors looked darkly in at him." So many nights in that drafty old farmhouse next door to Orrin's on Tilton Hill Road, nestled into my pocket of warmth beneath several hundred pounds of blankets, I listened to the same "roar of trees and crack of branches" the poem describes and puzzled over its final lines: "One aged man—one man—can't keep a house, / A farm, a countryside, or if he can, / It's thus he does it of a winter night."

Some time after his father died, Orrin sold his house and most of his lands to a neighbor who, like us, had come up from Massachusetts in the early 1960s. He kept one small field and a few acres of woods for himself but moved to a trailer park in Laconia. We didn't hear any more from him until several years later, when he began to return to our road—

to *his* road—to build himself a new house. He worked alone, on weekends and at odd hours, by now a man well into his 70s with a heart condition, building with his own hands the house in which he planned to live out his retirement. I saw him finish the house. I was home for Thanksgiving from college in Massachusetts, and Orrin Tilton was there every day that week, getting the roofing on before the first snow. By Sunday, he had got the roof on, and that afternoon in the early dusk, as I was driving away from our house, back to school, he had just finished splitting the winter's firewood. Actually, Orrin was leaving, too, headed back down to Laconia. His car stood in the road, blocking my way. As I waited for him to move, a neighbor came out of the nearby house (the daughter of the man who had bought Orrin's old house and land) and told me she had already called the police. By the time I got out and looked into his car, he was already gone: head sunk forward against the steering wheel, his face the color of parchment.

He had finished his house.

We stood with the blue lights of the police car flashing into the woods, a cold night coming on. I listened to branches crack and trunks creak, and the ground seemed to harden beneath my feet. I don't know what Orrin was feeling at the end, sitting in his car as the light failed. I suspect he had learned long before then what the poem tells us: that one man *can't* keep a house, a farm, a countryside, for as the psalm reminds us, "all things are transient, as insubstantial as dreams." And I suspect he also knew that if we *can* keep a house, it is through humble and ordinary acts such as hammering shingles and hauling wood, work performed not in a vain bid for immortality but out of plain reverence for the fact of being alive. His work was his worship, for such chores pay homage to the very impermanence of all we build. As Emerson writes, "in nature every moment is new; the past is always swallowed up and forgotten; the coming only is sacred. Nothing is secure but life, transition, the energizing spirit."

The old houses in our town were built to last, but the cellar holes in our woods remind us that houses, like bodies, don't endure forever. I don't know whether Orrin was religious or whether he would have been comforted by the apostle Paul's words: "we know that if the earthly house we live in is destroyed, we have a building from God, a house not made with hands, eternal in the heavens." Even those who don't believe in the afterlife described by Paul can share the feeling behind his words. On some level all religious feeling begins with the sense that our true home lies elsewhere, however we may choose to define *elsewhere*: as psychic wholeness; as life in the beloved community; as a place of justice; as a harmonious relation to the natural world; as union of our spirits with the Divine. In the journey to the elsewhere of our fond imagining we wish ourselves far from here, far from the suffering of our lives, far from our unfinished houses and our unfinished selves.

The unsettling news is that we'll never reach that elsewhere of our longing as long as we remain in this life, as long as we remain human. Heaven has its place, and our desire for it may guide us, ethically and spiritually, to work for the good. But in our desire always to be elsewhere than here, we can lose what measure of heaven may be ours on earth. When our fantasies of a better life consume us, when our memories of past hurts bind us and fears of pending calamity drive us, we are robbed of the only gift—the greatest gift—we can be sure of possessing: the present moment. We cannot summon the future, we cannot remake the past. The present moment is the unfinished house in which we dwell.

I don't know what awaits me after death: reincarnation as a houseplant or, if I've really racked up the bad karma, as a plastic surgeon in San Diego. Maybe the afterlife really *is* wings and harps and Mahalia Jackson, the Queen of Gospel, singing "In the Upper Room." Maybe it's nothing, absolutely nothing. I try not to make too much of those moments when I've had what Wordsworth called "intimations of immortality," when I have sensed the presence of another order of existence flickering like orange flames at the edges of the one I now know. Maybe these perceptions, and all religious feelings, are just delusional constructs that give the human species some evolutionary adaptive advantage by keeping us from annihilating one another even more efficiently than we do now. But I do know that whatever communion with the Divine I may have when this life is done will surely be prepared for by my seeking always to dwell in the Divine as I find it here, in this life, in this very moment. In each unfinished and imperfect day I struggle to find myself at home in this body, however flawed and failing, in this breath, however labored, in this speech, however halting. Each day, I work to make my home among the people I find about me. I write these words to make a sort of house in which you and I may dwell together for a time. Only in such work, in building a house of peace in the present moment, a house of peace not only for ourselves but for all who may be in our presence or our hearts—only in such work can we be made whole. We are here, in the unfinished house of the now, for the duration. The joy is in the building.

My mother eventually looked through the windows of enough farmhouses to want to sell our old one on Tilton Hill Road and move into a bigger, even older farmhouse on the other side of town. And a few years ago, my parents gave my wife and me the several acres of land on which we have built a house near theirs and in which we have the pleasure of hunkering through these long winter nights. Back when we were just starting to think about building, I was standing at a window in their house, looking out across the field to the section of dense woods where I was planning to build. It was a sub-zero December night, and the wind was up, lashing pines and blowing snow, the whole forest howling. I said to my mother then, "I can't imagine that we're really going to live out *there*." I suppose I was asking for her reassurance, and she gave it, saying simply, "You'll be fine." And we built the house, and we are fine, and I keep a file full of sketches for the addition, with its master bedroom and outdoor hot tub, its Count Rumford fireplace and radiant floor heat, its oak floors and cherry trim. And on some cold winter nights with the woodstove stoked I lie awake beside my wife and listen to "the roar of trees and crack of branches" that Frost described, and I'm thankful for the chance to be at home for this one night, for this one moment, in this unfinished house.

5

WILD THINGS

My dog has learned to hunt the mice that live beneath the snow. This is her first winter. She is a long, sleek, black affair, a mixture of various herding breeds, and lacking proper work she spends her days running the acres of our property, barking at trees, squirrels, and stones, barking at blue sky and clouds and wind, trying to gather her world together and move it toward some fitting destination. Her mouse hunting, too, is an elegant and futile business. With the snow frozen hard, she rears up on her hind legs and brings both front paws down together to punch through the crust. Sometimes she springs into the air to bring greater force to bear on her target. She then thrusts her snout into the hole to sniff out her prey. As far as I know she's never caught a thing. For a while we took all this frantic sniffing and punching and barking at the snow's blank white as just another form of canine folly. But then my eight-year-old son saw some coyotes on television hunting in the same way. So my dog's urge to punch snow must come from somewhere in the ancestral past she shares with her coyote cousins, a behavior uncoiled from some strand of doggie DNA. And when one night I watched a dark, thumb-sized blob of fuzz scoot over the snow before disappearing at the base of our bird feeder pole, I knew she was on to something after all. Once more, I was reminded how blind I am to the life around me, how unaware of the little things on which my world depends.

Among my town's mammals, after all, humans are a small minority, the thousand of us strung out like beads on the mostly dirt roads that thread our 100 square miles of forest, ledge and swamp. From the mountain peaks at the northern edge of town you can see little sign of human habitation. Roads, houses, and all but the largest fields are swallowed by trees, the white pinprick of the church steeple in the village center all that announces our presence to both God and the military fighter jets that practice maneuvers in our airspace. A friend of mine here used to say that he needed to hike these mountains once in a while in order to "get small," and you can see what he meant. From the vantage of these peaks, all the works of woman and man, the collective record of our striving, are a pinch of dust thrown on a carpet. That's probably just as well, for I find myself agreeing with Thoreau when he says that "a town is saved, not more by the righteous men [and women] in it than by the woods and swamps that surround it."

It's a good thing, too, that the animals in our midst seem to find us only a minor inconvenience. Oh, it's true that the animals sometimes inconvenience *us*, as when the moose lurches into the headlights' beam, an event common and dangerous enough to prompt the New Hampshire Fish and Game Department to put out a bumper sticker reading "Brake for Moose: It Could Save Your Life." Every neighborhood here has its bear, and I'm not the only one to have been awakened at dawn by the dull clang of my metal bird feeder pole being deftly bent to the ground. I suppose I should count it a privilege to descend the stairs in my robe and watch through glass as six feet away one happy adolescent omnivore sits on his haunches, the feeder tipped in his front paws like a tall glass of beer, pink tongue scouring the last seeds from the tube. And I do find it a privilege, as on a recent night, to step out into the cold air with moonlight shining on snow-covered fields and listen to coyotes sing from the edges of a frozen swamp. Wildness is all around us. Going into the woods after a snowfall, I'm startled to see the tracks—grouse, turkey, rabbit, squirrel, fox, ferret, beaver, bobcat—as though some sort of wildlife convention had been held while I slept. I hope one day to track the mountain lion a friend of mine saw bounding across a paved state road, its first leap taking it to the yellow center line, the next clear across into the woods where it disappeared once more into legend and the night fears of children.

Given the abundance of wild things around me, the wonder is that they remain for the most part as invisible as the mice beneath the snow. Sometimes it seems that we live surrounded by wildlife much the way some people believe themselves surrounded by angels. Wild things seem an entire order of life beyond the fringes of ordinary perception. My dog, reminding me coyote-fashion of this hidden realm, serves as a lesser angel, some intermediary spirit lower on the chain of being, linking me to the wild world. I have come to view her barking at the snow-covered ground as evidence of things unseen.

I'm being fanciful, of course, but not entirely. Let's remember that the word "animal" derives from the Latin *anima*, or "soul." To acknowledge one's own soul, then, is to acknowledge the animal within. And I would argue that to live consciously in the midst of wild things is to live in the midst of soul.

How might we understand and deepen our relationship to these two animal realms, these two soul realms, the wildness within and the wildness without? Thoreau wrote famously that "in Wildness is the preservation of the World." His disciple, John Muir, amended this as "in God's wildness lies the hope of the world." We see such words on Sierra Club calendars, as slogans urging us to preserve the wilderness. I'm less concerned here with land policy and wildlife management than with how we might have a deeper connection to wildness in our daily lives, how in becoming more fully wild we might preserve both our world and ourselves.

Mostly, we get the wrong idea about wildness. Some of our misuses of the term are innocent enough. As boys, hitting a home run in the back yard or sinking a long shot in the driveway hoop, we'd put on our best staticky sportscaster's voice to say "and the fans go WILD!" It was the nature of sports fans to go wild; indeed, going wild might even be the whole point of sports, which give us a time and place in which we can surrender to ecstasy. Sometimes by "going wild" we mean merely an impulsive and harmless loosening of restraints: when we try a daring new hair style or buy the black velvet dress *and* the lizard skin shoes. We get further off the track when we think of wildness as sexual excess, surrendering to primal impulses. When we think of this sort of wildness, of the "wild man" or "wild woman" in each of us, we think of fierce and passionate behavior that is both terrifying and alluring. To call someone an animal can be either a putdown, as in "you ANIMAL!" or a come-on, as in "you *animal,* you." We both desire such wildness and fear it. But we are furthest from the truth when we associate wildness with darkness and evil, where to go wild is to lose control, to give in to violence, to smash windows or bones.

It's no secret where wildness got this reputation. Since Plato and Aristotle we have seen reason as man's defining feature, what sets us apart from animals, and thus we become more human by becoming less animal. Just as biblical tradition grants us humans dominion "over all the wild animals of the earth," so the human reason of our minds has been granted dominion over the animal instincts of our bodies. We in the West have seen human nature not as an extension of animal nature but as at war against it, and have tried through much of our history to put as much distance as possible between our human and animal selves. Descartes went so far as to claim that animals were essentially machines, without mind, emotions, or souls, and therefore utterly different from us. Not until Freud did a Western thinker have the insight and the courage to argue that this denial of our animal natures makes us sick: as civilized men and women we may build great cities, but we will be unavoidably unhappy in them.

If we are to end our war with wildness we must learn to see it rightly. For our common notions of wildness—savage, ecstatic, excessive—have almost nothing to do with the actual wild creatures I see about me. Far from lacking control, the animals I know exemplify it. What you observe most often in wild animals is a quiet but purposeful awareness, an enviable sort of alert calm. Even the ruffed grouse, its brain the size of a Cheerio, steps and pecks past my cabin with greater assurance and self-discipline than shown by many folks I know even on their good days. More often than I like to think, I'd be willing to exchange my anxious, distracted state for that of the red squirrel, whose hectic scrabbling and foraging seems at least driven by a steady purpose and kinetic joy.

And savagery? Predators are fierce, but only as they need to be. Humans kill for sport; animals find sport in less violent pastimes. Predators, after all, spend far less time eating than do their foraging prey, and therefore they are noted layabouts. Lions laze, coyotes yodel, owls sleep late. The hawks that circle above my field are searching for prey, but much of the time they are simply soaring.

As for sex, here animals clearly have us beat. Almost all of them have the good sense to want it only at certain times of year. In other seasons they live free of the tormenting urges that account in one way or another for most of our gross national product. You would think, by the way, that with all our interest in sex we would enjoy it more than we do. As the poet Howard Nemerov puts it, "We think about sex obsessively except / During the act, when our minds tend to wander."

So wildness, rightly considered, has its advantages. On the other hand, I realize that living as an animal amounts to more than an extended camping trip. When I was a boy, watching deerflies crawl at the edges of a horse's eyes taught me something of the opportunities for misery this planet afforded. And I have hiked alone deep in grizzly bear country and felt what it was like to be part of the food chain. But somehow it was not until recently that I grasped the basic fact of animals' lives. It happened on one of those days that makes us New Englanders wonder why we don't move to Arizona: 33 degrees and driving sleet. I stood looking out the window at the woods, thinking of deer huddled beneath hemlocks, when suddenly it hit me: animals actually live *outdoors*. The moose that wander across our field, the deer that peep at us from the forest fringe are not on some sort of *outing*. They don't put in their appearances for us, then head back to the locker room for a shower and a change of clothes. Being an animal is a full-time occupation, hazardous and often brief: it's a sad truth that many animals live longer in captivity than they do in the wild.

So when I say that we should become more like wild things, I don't mean we should idealize them. We must avoid the Bambi syndrome, where all animals become wide-eyed innocents. Those mice tunneling beneath the snow sometimes eat their offspring. And any husband who says of his mate, "she'll chew my head off when I get home," should be glad he's not a male praying mantis, who suffers this fate quite literally during the most intimate of marital moments.

The prejudice that animals and nature are pure while humans and civilization are corrupt also has its own rich history. The French philosopher Jean Jacques Rousseau hatched the idea in the mid-eighteenth century, and from there it swam the English channel to seize the English Romantic poets, who in turn inspired Emerson and Thoreau, whose writings were tucked into John Muir's backpack on his rambles through Yosemite Valley, the accounts of which started modern environmentalism, a movement wherein the idea of nature's uncorrupted innocence flourishes today.

Fact is, animals are neither innocent nor guilty, neither pure nor corrupt, for these are strictly human categories. Indeed, if we're to envy animals, it's precisely because they live outside such categories. And here we come to the heart of the matter. For what would it mean to experience our own actions in such a way that the terms "good" and "bad" don't apply? It would mean living, like animals, without doubt as to our life's purpose. It would mean living in such perfect alignment with that purpose that our every act flowed effortlessly from what was highest and truest within us. It would mean rising each day to forage or feed, to shelter and care for our young, to laze or labor, fight or frolic without distraction, without self-judgment, without taking one step off life's true path. And even in the face of misery and terror, even as we walk through the valley of the shadow of death, even as the sleet freezes our hides or the hawk descends upon us, it would mean living in the faith that this, too, is the way. Imagine living in such fashion and you begin to imagine what I mean by becoming a wild thing.

But how to cultivate such a life? Perhaps I'm not the one to try to answer such a question. These days as my body weakens I have a hard enough time getting my shirt on in the morning without questioning my life's purpose, without falling prey to the fear and self-judgment that lie in wait for all of us thinking animals, just around the bend from each happy thought. Tottering on the stairs, laboring a quarter of an hour to spread cream cheese on a bagel, I find myself moaning along with William Butler Yeats as he laments his aging body:

What shall I do with this absurdity—
O heart, O troubled heart—this caricature,
Decrepit age that has been tied to me
As to a dog's tail?

I could console myself by thinking that some of my life's purpose these days is fulfilled by my writing. In my more grandiose moods I might even imagine that some of my words will live on after my death. Such moments pass, however, and I find myself siding with Woody Allen when he says, "I don't want to attain immortality through my work. I want to attain immortality by not dying."

So if I say that I'm learning to be a wild thing, you must understand that even on my best days I am not nearly so wild as I would like. Still, one must make the effort, and I will say that it is in the state of wildness, however fleeting, that I find what peace my days afford. But first things first: cultivating your own wildness, as much as pole vaulting or the French horn, takes practice. That is, you must first *have* a practice, and then you must practice it. There are many forms such practice can take, but all require that we set aside some part of each day for solitude and silence. For some this takes the form of meditation or prayer, for others long distance running does the trick; it could be sitting or walking in the out of doors, or it could be quiet and mindful absorption in a simple task such as knitting or making bread.

By this sort of practice I don't mean reflection, I don't mean soul-searching or analysis or deliberation. In fact, I don't mean *thinking* of any kind. Our problem, after all, is that we think *too much*. Thinking has its place, but at some point it becomes a means of avoiding our lives instead of living them. We're after what the jazz great Bill Evans found in common between Japanese ink brush painting and musical improvisation. Each brush stroke, like each note played, cannot be rehearsed, and once laid down, cannot be undone. "Direct deed," he writes, "is the most meaningful reflection." In our practice of wildness, as in artistic improvisation, as in life, we must bring all our experience and skill to bear, but what matters most is that we do only the task at hand, that we give ourselves fully to the moment. So in your practice don't meditate to think about your life, don't go running to plan your next career move, don't knit to do something useful while you watch TV. There is nothing wrong, of course, with doing any of these things, but we should not confuse them with the practice of wildness.

An accomplished Indian yogi said that "self-observation without judgment is the highest spiritual discipline." It's this quality of awareness, what some call "witness consciousness," that we are after. Both the method and the goal of practice are to be fully present to the moment and to ourselves in an attitude of total self-acceptance.

Wild animals, of course, don't have to accept themselves. They can simply *be*. As *thinking* animals, we must work to create some space for our wild natures, to give them room to roam. Whether keeping our awareness on the breath as we meditate, on our bodies' rhythm as we run, on our sensations as we sink our hands in bread dough, our practice anchors us in our bodies, takes us further into our wild selves. With time (months, years, decades, lifetimes—did you think this would be easy?) such practice begins to open a space within us. Call it a wildlife preserve, a space where our wild selves can breathe while our judging, criticizing, worrying, doubting minds are kept safely on the other side of the fence. With practice we find ourselves living more and more inside this preserve, a place we come to recognize as our true home.

Our minds, of course, will continue to stand outside the fence, sharing their opinions with us. There you are: you've lit your candles, burned your incense, said your mantra, and now you find yourself in your wildlife preserve. Maybe it's open savanna, a tree-dotted plain with animals grazing, and you find yourself seated beneath a shade tree, a breeze cooling your brow, everything at peace, and meanwhile there's your other self, your human, civilized self, the one with the sweaty palms, the one with the *agenda,* standing not far off behind the fence saying, "you're not doing this *right,* you know." You've punched down your bread dough and are reshaping the loaf, and there's your mind whispering, "your mother-in-law makes better bread." You're into mile four of your run, getting your stride, feeling good, and from outside the fence a voice points out that you should have bought the other running suit, the less revealing one, because right now there are people scheduling meetings to discuss your thighs.

This is what the mind *does,* after all. Like my dog who spends her days yapping at snow and trees and sky, the mind wants to feel useful. We cannot silence these voices—they, too, deserve our compassionate acceptance. We can, however, move the fence a little further out, gradually claiming more ground for our wildness, until the voices are not so loud, their breath not so hot in our ears.

Thoreau said that "the most alive is the wildest." We don't go into wildness to escape our lives but to return to them, to return to our true selves and our highest purposes. In wildness we live out the Christian injunction to "be in the world but not of it." We find ourselves, as Walt Whitman, "both in and out of the game."

For let's remember that practice is just that: practice for the rest of our lives. We do not meditate or run or make bread merely to claim an hour's calm from the day's calamity— though that in itself has great value. We practice so that we may bring some part of that calm into the remaining hours of the day. We practice wildness so that we may live more fully and constantly in the midst of *anima,* in the midst of soul. When I have claimed my wildness I can find myself, with Whitman, "aplomb in the midst of irrational things." Wildness will not save us from misfortune. Fear, doubt, grief all lie in wait to strike and seize us as before. Only now their grip will not be so tight or last so long. In life's thicket we will have created a clearing for our wild selves. And in that clearing, in the face of confusion and worry, in the face of failure and loss, in the face of death itself, we will lift our noses to the moon and sing.

6

OUT OF THE CAVE

In the first week of April, the wood frogs in our neighborhood scrabble out of whatever muck they winter in and gather at the vernal pool in the woods below our house. Though ice still skins one end of the pool, the frogs are loudly sociable, and for two weeks, as I sit writing in my cabin fifty yards off, their raucous quacking is my daily music. In the two months between its forming and its drying up, this shallow pool is a busy place. In the second week of April, the peepers begin their nighttime trilling; tree frogs, leopard frogs, and green frogs wait their turns. On rainy nights spotted salamanders crawl from beneath rotting logs and make their way there to breed in writhing heaps. As the tadpoles fatten, turtles will claw out of streams and ponds as much as a mile away and travel here to eat them. Raccoon, ferret, and fox venture from their dens to gobble frogs. All around us life unburies itself.

Every few days my children and I take a bucket and net into the woods to check the pool's progress. Seeing animals has proven difficult: our clumsy approach sends the frogs diving beneath the leaves at the bottom. On our first visits we see no sign that all this amphibian mingling had come to much, but at last my son dips a bucketful of ale-colored water and finds the payoff: tadpoles no bigger than seeds in rye bread.

Looking carefully, we also find squiggling insect larvae, tiny paddling beetles, assorted scooters, blobs and bumblers we don't know the names of. There's even more we cannot see: all the microscopic floaters and crawlers, the paramecia and bacteria, the broad and invisible base of that great food pyramid at whose pinnacle my children and I are improbably perched.

Bending over the bucket, peering past my reflection on the water's stilled surface, I find myself thinking that, first and last, life consists of eating and being eaten. If somewhere along the way we manage to reproduce, so much the better. Food and sex: what else animates us? Ads for Caribbean vacations, featuring tanned flesh and heaped platters, tempt us to spend a week—and a lot of money—thinking of nothing else.

But other pleasures, mainly social ones, pull us into the company of others, especially at this time of year. The frogs' spring ritual is a collective one, and spring pulls us humans, too, out of our winter hidey holes. Even the most harried suburban commuter lingers in the morning sun between house and automobile, scouting for crocuses. On weekends we unbend our winter postures with yard work, hailing neighbors not sighted during the dark months. In our town, where most of us have no neighbors within hailing distance, the urge to see people takes us into the village, where a trip to the post office and general store becomes an hour's social adventure. Traveling a few hundred yards I am greeted by a dozen people. A friend stops her car in the street; I stand on the yellow center line, talking through the rolled down window. Our frail elderly, counting their losses and their blessings, emerge from their houses blinking to greet us in the light of one more spring. We stand in the street holding mail, newspapers, coffee, glad to be alive in that rejuvenating air.

On such days I'm happy to come out of my cave, and am reminded of the enlivening force of community. This winter

I've spent a good part of most days alone in my 10-by-12 cabin, meditating, reading, and writing. So much of spiritual life involves one's interior journey, yet for most of us spirituality gets expressed—even transformed—only in our relationships with others.

Granted, we have to take time out from our routine busyness to develop—and bring to the rest of our days' activities—that state of calm, alert, awareness one observes in animals, whose every action seems to flow effortlessly from their true natures. But most animals, and especially humans, don't live alone. Our relationships with others not only test our spiritual resources, but push us to levels of development we could not attain through solitary practice.

More important, our gifts to others are the very fruits of our own self-development. The two forms of life, communal and solitary, are mutually sustaining. Even the Christian Desert Fathers, those fourth-century hermits who sought extreme solitude in the Egyptian desert, understood that simply running away from society would serve no purpose. When one of them told another of his plans to "shut himself into his cell and refuse the face of men, that he might perfect himself," the second monk replied that "unless thou first amend thy life going to and fro amongst men, thou shall not avail to amend it dwelling alone." These ancient seekers, practicing disciplines unimaginably severe to our coddled sensibilities, grasped a truth lost amid the heaps of self-help books and rarely heard within the walls of the therapist's office: seeking only our *own* happiness is the surest way to remain unhappy. As the great monastic and scholar Thomas Merton puts it, "Isolation in the self, inability to go out of oneself to others, would mean incapacity for any form of self-transcendence. To be thus the prisoner of one's own selfhood is, in fact, to be in hell."

Most of us know this. Even if we're drawn to the spiritual life and feel the pull of solitude, few of us these days wish to be hermits. We want our solitude, but we also want to raise families, pursue careers, take part in the wider world, and make a difference to others. Perhaps we're after what was known in Latin as the *vita mixta*, the mixed life of action and contemplation in which, as St. Augustine says, "the love of truth doth ask a holy quiet, and the necessity of love doth accept a righteous busyness." Lest self-development become self-enclosure and stagnation, we must leave the cave and enter the light of relationship, family, and community. If we accept what all the world religions tell us, that on the deepest levels our separateness from others is an illusion, then our own spiritual self-fulfillment is intimately bound to the fulfillment of those around us. A rising tide lifts all boats, and each of us empties his or her own cup into the ocean of spirit. This truth is grasped by the people whom the Buddhists call Bodhisattvas, who refuse the rewards of their own enlightenment in order to work for the enlightenment of all other beings. In this view, we get to heaven together or not at all. Speaking from the standpoint of the self-enclosed, alienated individual, Jean-Paul Sartre wrote famously that "hell is other people." Yet when we leave the cave in a spirit of true selflessness, we find just the opposite: other people are heaven itself, the place of our full realization as human beings.

But it's easy, you might say, for me to wax ecstatic about other people from my solitary cabin in the woods. The only thing hanging on the wall of my cabin is a topographical map of the region, actually four such maps cut and pasted together on a piece of cardboard. It's a homely but useful construction, some forty years old, rescued from my parents' attic. Consulting it, and adding the houses built in the four decades since the map was drawn, I see that within a one-mile radius of where I write most mornings there are at most six humans other than me. I know them all by name. Later, when people come home from work, the number grows, to 15 perhaps. Five belong to my immediate family. I go for days at a time without riding in an automobile or seeing anyone I do not know well. What, you might ask, could such a person possibly have to tell you about living in community?

I would answer that nothing serves relationships, families, or communities better than a well-cultivated solitude. Of course, solitude has never been fashionable. We are not bears, after all, but primates, bound to the intricate and noisy life of the troupe. Among humans, solitaries have always excited suspicion and ridicule. Once I told a woman I had just started dating that I was going to spend several days at a Benedictine monastery, living in a cave in the bluffs overlooking the Mississippi river. By the look the woman gave me, it was clear she figured me for a lost cause, if not outright dangerous in some way she couldn't quite define.

Now that we've been married for 13 years, she has learned to tolerate my need for solitude. As it turns out, she has the same need herself, and perhaps what she really feared then was that neither one of us would be very good at managing a household. In fact, we're both good at it—better, I would argue, for having practiced the arts of solitude. Having given generously and fully to ourselves, we can give generously and fully to each another and our children and, by extension, to our communities.

The Chinese *I Ching*, or *Book of Changes*, teaches that "A healthy family, a healthy country, a healthy world—all grow outward from a single superior person" and therefore directs us to "begin by improving ourselves." But becoming a superior person sometimes requires more discipline than even the best of us can muster. For one thing, the *vita mixta* requires equal attention to both action and contemplation. Augustine's "righteous busyness" must be founded upon times of "holy quiet." Without replenishing ourselves with solitude, we will find that our busyness—all our doing and giving and caring—leaves us only frustrated, resentful, and exhausted. "It is so easy to simply get too busy to grow," writes the Benedictine monastic Joan Chittister. "It is so easy to commit ourselves to this century's demand for product and action until the product consumes us and the actions exhaust us and we can no longer even remember why we set out to do them in the first place." Worse, without holy quiet, righteous busyness easily becomes *self*-righteous. We've all caught ourselves at times when our efforts to do good in the world—to teach our children, help our communities, correct an injustice—have more to do with looking good or proving something than with a genuine, selfless desire to serve. Thomas Merton warns us that "he who attempts to act and do things for others or for the world without deepening his own self-understanding, freedom, integrity and capacity to love, will not have anything to give to others. He will communicate to them nothing but the contagion of his own obsessions, his aggressiveness, his ego-centered ambitions, his delusions about ends and means, his doctrinaire prejudices and ideas." And for Merton, the Cistercian monk, deepening one's own self-understanding requires a disciplined practice of meditation or contemplative prayer, made possible only by regular doses of holy quiet.

Now, I don't know what your household is like, but my wife and I find that, between making a living and raising two young children, holy quiet is hard to come by. Sometimes holy hell is more like it. The dog has just muddied the sofa, my son refuses my 14th polite request to pick up his Legos from the floor where I'm walking, at great peril to my neck, trying to get the table set for dinner. My daughter begins screaming that she *hates* the butterfly she's just painted and now she's *ruined* the watercolor for Grandma's birthday she's been working on for the past half-hour, with its flowers and tree and rainbow and smiling sun. My wife and I insist that it's a *beautiful* painting and Grandma won't even notice the butterfly, which is, we admit, a bit crumpled and deformed-looking. Our lovely daughter screams louder. Meanwhile the house fills with smoke from the fish left unattended in the broiler, giving my wife and I time to exchange only one mutually accusatory glance before the smoke alarm has us all holding our hands over our ears wondering why God has had to go so Old Testament on us all of a sudden and just what will be the extent of His wrath.

Driving to work, or even a trip to the supermarket, can seem a blessed escape from the teeming, dense life of the family. Soon enough, though, we find that we are no more superior outside of the home than within it. Far from joyfully embracing our connectedness with our fellow-divine-beings-clothed-in-human-form, we spend our days artfully evading any genuine contact with them. In the supermarket you spot an acquaintance—the one with the grating laugh and the habit of bragging about her children—and you discover a sudden interest in the Pet Supplies aisle, even though Fluffy died three years ago. At work you see a colleague approaching in the hall—for three weeks now you've owed him that memo on forming a committee to coordinate the efforts of interdepartmental coordinating committees—and you look for a doorway to duck into. When we do let people get close enough to open their mouths in our presence, we do anything but actually listen to them. We judge, we analyze, we defend, we recall the 3.2 times each week, on average, that this person has said this same thing for the past year now, and we wonder how many more times we'll have to hear it before one of us moves to the Orkney Islands to raise sheep.

No wonder, then, that at the end of the day it's such a relief to get home. Only when we get there do we remember that it's the people we live with we are most desperate to avoid. Funny how I can miss my wife terribly all day until the moment I walk in the house. We have a wonderful marriage, but some days it seems that the whole point of long-term relationships is to give people time to learn to torment one another efficiently. We become athletes of insult, proud of our ability not just to inflict pain, but to do so with minimum effort. We know a relationship is fully developed when with a single lifted eyebrow we can ruin someone's entire day.

Estranged from others outside the house and finding no holy quiet within it, we go into the cave to seek the holy quiet of solitude. But we must be careful not to think of our retreat into the cave as an escape, for the demons that beset us in our lives outside the cave will surely follow us into it. The abbot Antony, one of the earliest and greatest of the Desert Fathers, reminds us, "Who sits in solitude and is quiet hath escaped from three wars: hearing, speaking, seeing: yet against one thing shall he continually battle: that is, his own heart." We must go into the cave, then, not to escape our lives but to go more fully into them, to dwell with deeper awareness and acceptance of all we are and all that befalls us.

A friend of mine, a sculptor who works in steel, says, "I have to spend a certain amount of my time alone in my studio, or I can't stand to be with people." When I asked whether he did this to escape, he answered, "It's about seeking self-understanding." By self-understanding he does not mean self-analysis. My friend does not go into his studio to think about himself or his life. He goes there to cut, bend, weld, and grind metal (the Desert Fathers wove baskets of palm leaves), and through mindful absorption in this work to empty himself, for a time, of the daily demands and petty assertions of his ego. Nor is going into the cave about creating some *product:* my friend makes no great effort to sell his work; the Desert Fathers sold their baskets and gave the money to the poor. To go into the cave to *accomplish* something—even self-understanding, even enlightenment—is to risk falling back into the trap that the ego lays just ahead of all our best intentions. As the thirteenth-century Sufi mystic and poet, Jalal al-Din Rumi, reminds us, "No better love than love with no object, / no more satisfying work than work with no purpose."

You may already have your own way of going into the cave. It may be prayer or gardening or yoga or long distance running. There are plenty of books and courses teaching meditation from within Buddhist, Hindu, and Christian traditions. I'm not concerned with technique so much as attitude. Though regularity and discipline matter, spiritual practice is not simply about observing routines and rituals. Yoga can be a spiritual practice or just another fitness regimen. You can carve wood to cultivate mindful awareness or to produce duck decoys. As the Buddhist monk Thich Nhat Hanh says, "There are two ways to wash the dishes. The first is to wash the dishes in order to have clean dishes and the second is to wash the dishes in order to wash the dishes." Only the second way—washing the dishes in order to wash the dishes—constitutes a spiritual practice.

We enter the cave only when we dwell fully, mindfully in the present moment. We enter the cave only when we are willing to empty ourselves of all that our ordinary, busy selves hold most dear: our plans, our ambitions, our intelligence, our precious opinions, our hard won expertise, our reputations, everything within us that desires a reward, a purpose, an end. In this emptying, this letting go, we make room for something else. We allow ourselves to be entered and filled with that essential goodness that is our surest inheritance. We become more deeply and consciously connected to what is highest and truest within us. We dwell more fully in contact with the Divine. When we leave the cave replenished with this goodness, made whole again by this contact with our higher nature, we find ourselves less fearful, more willing to venture ourselves for the good. Conflicts disappear, relationships blossom, communities prosper, love grows.

I know this isn't easy. Often my idea of going into the cave is turning on the basketball game and ordering out for pizza. On such days I can't summon the energy or courage to face myself—or others. One of Meister Eckhart's many enigmatic sayings is that "God's exit is his entrance." He also says that "to the extent that all creatures who are gifted with reason go out from themselves in all that they do, to that same extent they go into themselves." That is, when I truly go out of myself in meeting another person, when in that encounter I can let go of my small, fearful, grasping self, then in meeting the other I simultaneously meet my own highest, truest self. If each individual being is an outflowing from— and point of access into—the same divine source that flows through all (call this source God, Life, Love, Brahman, Being, High Self, Spirit, or what you will), then in opening myself to another's essential nature I am at the same time opening myself to my own. The biblical commandment to "love thy neighbor as thyself" is in this light transformed from a moral rule to a profound statement about the nature of relationship. I can love another only as I love myself. Conversely, I can love myself only as I love another. Love's exit is its entrance. We see others as strangers only when we are estranged from ourselves. We can fear in others only what we fear in ourselves. And when we meet a loved one, we are meeting ourselves as the beloved.

We all know the difference between managing a conflict and dissolving one. We manage a conflict through discussion and analysis. We gather the facts, assess one another's needs, make lists, divide responsibilities: I'll put the laundry in the washing machine, you transfer it to the dryer, I'll fold it, you put it away. We've all made these arrangements. But we have also known those moments when the need for analysis, arrangements, and lists melts away, when conflict dissolves like sugar in tea. It's in those moments that we go out of ourselves, and simultaneously go into ourselves, into our own essential goodness. At such moments we surrender all advantages, give up all claims to righteousness, relinquish all privileges except that of being in the presence—the sacred and unfathomable presence—of another.

A traditional greeting among Indian Hindus is *namaste*

(nama-STAY), said with a slight bow, palms pressed together in front of the heart. Literally it means, "I bow to you" or "I salute you," and to an Indian is simply a respectful way of saying hello. Understood within its religious context, however, the greeting acknowledges that the other person is, like oneself, an individual manifestation of Brahman, the sacred essence of all created things. *Namaste* can be translated more fully, then, as "I bow to the life spirit within you that is also within me." What a lovely way to greet people! I don't often do it, for fear they'll question my sanity, yet upon meeting someone I often say this greeting silently to myself. It's especially useful when meeting someone I ordinarily find wearisome, difficult, or threatening. The shift can be remarkable. One moment we're doing what we usually do when someone speaks to us: we're judging, defending, analyzing, etc.. The next moment we are actually listening. Our angry, judgmental, impatient voice doesn't ever go away, of course. With practice, though, you can tune it out—if not forever then at least for long enough to greet the person rolling her shopping cart toward you now, the person with the expensive hair and neurotic high-achieving children, the one whom a moment ago you would have avoided by diving into Pet Supplies, but who now approaches you transformed, face alight with friendship, offering you in her welcoming smile a better version of yourself than you thought you possessed.

I don't mean to sound naive. There are some people we rightfully avoid, and we need not feel guilty about that. As someone is coming toward me with a knife, I'm not trying to accept the knife-wielder within me. And if someone has harmed me, it is right to forgive but not forget and to take appropriate measures to avoid such harm in the future.

When asked about the problem of responding to violence, the Dalai Lama of Tibet replied, "Tolerance and patience do not imply submission or giving in to injustice." What is most important, he says, is not to give in to anger or hatred. If we cannot control others' actions, we can control our responses to them. Sopa, the Tibetan word for patience, comes from a root that means "able to withstand." The truly courageous person, says the Dalai Lama, is able to withstand harm without the mental suffering that hatred and anger bring.

The violence I suffer every day is the slow, niggling kind committed by a degenerative illness bent on emptying me out one teaspoon at a time. Every day, I relearn that suffering is an activity of the mind. My hours fill with torment or bliss depending on my own degree of *sopa*, my ability to withstand physical harm while maintaining an inner calm. It's like learning to relax in the dentist's chair: if you could practice during every waking moment you might get good at it.

But my illness is just a particular form of the universal human malady. We all suffer the limitations of our humanness: not just our aches and pains, but our fear, our anger, our pettiness, our grief. Fact is, we *do* practice being human in every waking moment. And the more mindfully we practice, the more often our conflicts dissolve, the more easily we create new possibilities for relationship and community.

On a recent evening I attended my son's and daughter's first piano recital, a kind of event I normally dread. Children, parents, and grandparents packed the small old church in the village center. Amelia, at age six the youngest performer on the program, had to go first, and I endured a stretch of terror watching her march solemnly to the front, climb onto the piano bench, and play a flawless rendition of that immortal classic, "Fuzzy Baby Bird."

It turned out to be a wonderful recital. Amelia and Aaron played well, but more to my surprise, so did everyone else, and we were treated to what I had least expected: an evening of good music. Still, in the midst of it, I found myself growing sad. With my weakened and trembling hands I can no longer play the piano or the guitar as I once did, and the more beautiful the music I heard that night, the more keenly I felt the loss. I knew such feelings came from what the Zen Buddhists call "small mind," from my grasping, fearful self, unable to let go and simply enjoy the moment. So I took heart, thinking that at least *someone* was playing, that these children were carrying on where I no longer could.

But then something more happened, something I can barely put into words. All of a sudden it was as though I *were* playing the piano but playing through these children. Only it was no longer a matter of "me" and "them." *We* were playing the piano. For a few moments I broke through into what is called "big mind," that state of being in which the illusion of our separateness falls away, when our attachments dissolve, and we experience the boundlessness of our true nature.

Over the years, the more regularly I have gone into the cave, the more often I have these moments of big mind, and indeed the more ordinary they have become. I find myself challenged to imagine what human relationship and community could be like were we to live in such a state always. I imagine living more nearly as animals do, without either the blessing or the burden of self-awareness. What music we could make! I imagine us as frogs in our pool in the woods. Unburdened of self, we have just crawled from the muck and for one purpose only: to announce our amorous intent, our collective call to love.

7

MUD SEASON

I undertook my first road improvement project at age six or seven, removing the pebbles from the dirt road in front of our house. It was the work of an idle summer afternoon: I dug stones out of packed dirt and flung them into a field. I felt I was acting for the general welfare and planned on telling my parents that evening at dinner about the good I'd done in smoothing the road. But then my father came out and told me to stop. We needed those stones in the road, he told me. This made no sense: wasn't it better to make the road smooth? No, he explained, the stones made the road hard. We needed a hard road more than a smooth one.

It took me many years to understand what my father meant. In some ways, I'm still learning. There's geology to consider. New Hampshire is the Granite State and at bottom our town is a rumpled bed of stone scoured clean by glaciers that withdrew only 10,000 years ago. Ice still haunts us: you can hike into these mountains in the heat of summer, peer into a deep stone crevice and find it there, pale and dirty, its chill breath seeming to whisper all we'll ever know of endurance: *I was, I am, I will be.* The prolonged violence of the glaciers' melting notched our valleys and piled up gravel, those round river stones I spent a childhood summer afternoon flinging into the field. After the melt, life took hold, and eventually trees, but a hundred centuries of death and resurrection have yielded only a meager soil, laid like a thin sponge over that unyielding granite bed. With the March thaw, that sponge sops full: streams gush, swamps rise, bogs flush, forest hollows fill with vernal pools. For several weeks, with snow still knee deep in shadowed woods and on the north sides of buildings, we live in a between time, neither winter nor spring. No hymns are written in its praise. It's a time of neither here nor there, a non-season when, as T.S. Eliot wrote, "between melting and freezing / the soul's sap quivers." The literal sap quivers in the maples, drawn off in buckets and boiled for syrup, but this is the season's only sweetness. Mostly it's the season of mud.

In March and early April in our town, over 70 miles of dirt roads turn to mud, and most of our driveways, too. Paved roads are too expensive for us; we are simply too few and far flung. And paved driveways are shunned as being too suburban even by those who can afford them. Our road agent patrols with the town's police chief, posting Day-Glo signs declaring some roads officially closed due to mud. In theory, that's to save the town crews the trouble of rescuing vehicles sunk to their axles—though every year they have to haul a few out anyway. Mud coats the flanks of our cars, splatters our clothes, cakes our shoes. Children here, of course, are mud connoisseurs. In their school art classes my kids are handed sponges and brown paint and told to do paintings of mud. After school, I meet them where the bus drops them out on the paved state road, and we walk home through the real thing. We stomp and squish, we poke and stir, we sample textures and colors. Sometimes it takes us nearly an hour to walk the quarter mile. Children, so much closer to the source of life, seem in touch with their muddy origins. From dust you came, the priests used tell me, thumbing my forehead with ashes. Dust, yes, but for there to be life you have to add water, and we know what that makes.

Mud even figures in our architecture: houses here have an entire room devoted to it. When we finally reach home, my children and I leave boots and coats in the mud room, and sometimes pants and socks, too, so that we often enter our dwelling half naked but mud-free. Except for the dog, who doesn't understand mud rooms, and must be chased down with the towel we keep by the door.

Mud season brings portents. Buds swell: already a blush appears in the red maples above the swamp. Daffodils poke up from the earth, only to be buried by a late snowfall. A coyote limps across our field in full day. Jesus rides a donkey into Jerusalem, knowing that men wait there to kill him. Our minds cannot grasp the coming change: in three months I'll plunge my body into the same lake I walked across only weeks ago.

Mostly we fear it, this loosening of winter's hold, the shedding of ice certainties. We fear this time of year not so much for where it's taking us—the spring bloom and summer roar—but for what we have to go through to get there. We've all heard that Christmas is the busiest season for suicides, but I've heard that in New England it's mud season. Mud stirs dangerous longings and reminds us of all we'd prefer to forget. The entire direction of civilization is away from mud. We measure our progress with pavement. The modern city or suburb, with its paved streets and sidewalks, its curbs and storm drains, is really a giant mud avoidance system, designed at great expense to lift us into higher and drier versions of ourselves. The word *pavement* derives from the Latin *pavire*, to stamp or beat, and indeed we try to beat down our muddy origins and muddy selves, to suppress all things untoward and unseemly, to make our way smooth. But here in March, on roads laid more lightly over the land, pavement heaves and buckles, as though after winter's iron months a terrible secret strains to surface.

We all, of course, go through personal mud seasons, and these can occur at any time of year. We suffer illness and depression, the loss of loved ones, failed or failing marriages, crises of faith—in ourselves, in others, in our gods. But personal mud seasons need not be brought on by things so great as these. Humans have a peculiar talent for misery, and lacking big reasons for unhappiness, we make ingenious use of small ones, all the bounced-check and runny-nose occasions of woe. We need the mud, it seems, for our mud seasons give us the pleasure of self-pity, which for most of us ranks between bowling and sex. Now, my illness weakens certain parts of the body but not others, and I'm sorry to say I've had to give up bowling. (I guess that's okay: though sex doesn't last as long as bowling, you can do it without having to rent funny shoes.)

Still, having given up certain pleasures, I must pursue the ones that remain to me more often, including the pleasure of self-pity. I've needed mud more than ever, and a fatal illness offers the advantage of keeping mud close at hand. A few short, wobbly steps have me wallowing. But it's been five years now, and as a source of mud my illness has lost its freshness. Even the glamour of tragedy wears thin, and I must fall back on the ordinary, everyday returns to mud we all so much depend upon: my computer crashes, the dog chews the window sill, my children cut each other's hair with poultry shears, my wife fails to appreciate my talent for staring out the window at the bird feeder. Mud, mud, mud.

I've learned, though, that our need for mud goes much deeper than our need to pity ourselves. We need the mud for what grows from it. Every mud season is a kind of death, with resurrection lying on the other side. In the mud painting my daughter did at school, the great brown swath across the bottom two-thirds of the paper is topped with tiny, bright flowers. The image suggests causality—mud makes flowers—

but also necessity: no mud, no flowers. As I enter my various mud seasons, I've learned to ask: what death is this? Or what is it within me that needs to die? And out of this death, what resurrection will come?

My thoughts return to that Jewish peasant riding a borrowed donkey into Jerusalem the week before Passover. Reading that people laid branches and spread their cloaks on the road before him, the New Englander can conclude only one thing: he was riding through mud. What can this man teach me about going through the mud, about dying and being raised up?

There's so much the nuns never taught me. Maybe I just wasn't paying attention, but it seems I had to grow to adulthood to figure out that Christ wasn't a last name, like Harper or Hassan, but a descriptive title: Jesus the Christ, Jesus the anointed one. Anointed in what sense? For answers to this question I've been turning lately to voices I didn't hear in childhood. In recent years the work of such biblical scholars as John Crossan and Marcus Borg has taught us much about the historical Jesus, including the political and social context of his teachings and actions. Their work has also helped me get a feel for Jesus as a man. The Jesus of my childhood was a willowy, doe-eyed figure who spent too much time in his bathrobe. I liked his ideas—turning the other cheek and loving your enemy seemed both difficult and deeply right—but Jesus himself was strange and unappealing. I was told that he loved me and that I should love him back, but for a child love lies close to the skin, a matter of texture and heat: my father's scratchy face, my mother's soft arms. I didn't see how I could love someone so remote as this Jesus in heaven.

It was through reading literature that I eventually learned to love people I had never met and who may not even have existed. We call these people characters, and I think I know enough of Jesus now to see him as a great character in the most dramatic of situations.

The scene is Jerusalem, a Jewish city under a brutal Roman occupation. It's the week before Passover, and for days Jewish peasants have streamed into the city from the surrounding countryside, preparing to celebrate at the Temple. Their presence makes the Roman authorities nervous. Recent years have seen a string of apocalyptic prophets leading peasant uprisings; the Romans have had to kill them and their followers by the thousands. Now word is out that another troublemaker, this man Jesus from Galilee, is on his way. There's a buzz among the peasants thronging the Temple precincts. The Roman authorities and their collaborators among the city's Jewish aristocracy, including the scribes and Pharisees, can only watch and wait for their moment.

And here comes Jesus, astride his donkey, slogging though mud, with a crowd of followers around him and more people coming out to meet him on the road. In my version, the twelve disciples are men under those robes, and Jesus has chest hair. But there are women, too: Mary Magdalene, a person of high spiritual attainment, walks confidently at his side. People are calling out to him on every side: prayers, praise, requests for healing. Jesus knows the Pharisees among the crowd are watching him closely, waiting for him to slip up. He knows they would just as soon see him dead.

Then some of the Pharisees, alarmed by the crowd's enthusiasm, call out, "Teacher, order your disciples to stop." At this point a lesser man would make some ingratiating or politic reply. But Jesus answers: "I tell you, if these were silent, the stones would shout out."

Now, this is a man I can love. I imagine him speaking these words not with haughtiness or pride, but out of a calm conviction of the rightness of his actions. In mud season all the land cries out the coming change, and Jesus felt himself so aligned with the natural and cosmic order that the very stones would cry out his arrival. Jesus at this moment is in the state of true wildness, when we express our divine natures as effortlessly as animals do, when our every word and deed flows directly from our highest purposes. It's in this same state of wildness that he later clears the Temple, and ultimately goes to his death. How would this world be transformed if we could all go to our deaths with such clarity of conviction? How would my life be transformed if I could go to my death in such sure faith? What new life would wake within me if I could slog through the mud of my passage here—through my great trials and everyday afflictions—with the grace and courage of this man?

Wishing that we could live like Jesus may be too much to ask. On most days if I manage to keep my shirt tucked in and refrain from kicking the dog, I figure I've made my spiritual progress for the day. And when we do hanker for moral uplift, we know it's easier to seek inspiration from men and women nearer to us. In our schools we justly celebrate the lives of such secular saints as Harriet Tubman and Martin Luther King Jr., figures less problematic because certifiably mortal. True religion is an activity of the imagination, and perhaps Jesus remains impossible to imagine afresh, buried as he is beneath centuries of cultural myth and the accumulated debris of our religious upbringings, Christian or not, happy or not. But as someone who wandered from his Catholic upbringing to follow other paths—Buddhist and Hindu spiritual practices, intramural basketball, and reading poetry while drinking café latte—I find myself returning by odd and circuitous routes to this dual figure of Jesus the man and Jesus the Christ. And hard as it may be, if I want to love Jesus the man, the peasant revolutionary and visionary radical, I must also come to terms with Jesus the Christ, Jesus the anointed one, a figure who is something more than a man. But how to do this?

Again I listen for voices I didn't hear in my childhood. For example, I rediscover Jesus in the words of His Holiness the Dalai Lama of Tibet, who recognizes Jesus as either a fully enlightened being or as a bodhisattva, a person of high spiritual attainment who has chosen to remain in the cycle of birth and death to help others find their way to enlightenment (see *The Good Heart: A Buddhist Perspective on the Teachings of Jesus*). I rediscover Jesus as the man Islamic people revere as a great prophet and saint, and as the mysterious and powerful figure who rides through the poems of the great Sufi mystic Jalal al-Din Rumi. I rediscover Jesus in the writings of the medieval Christian mystic Meister Eckhart, who if asked whether Jesus was God's only begotten son, would answer: "Yes, and so am I, and so are you." Hearing these and other voices, I imagine Jesus the man as one of God's many embodiments in the world, and I imagine Jesus the Christ as that potential divinity within each of us. When we enter into that which is divine within us, we enter our own Christhood, our own Christ-consciousness. To stand fully within that presence, to live and move in such alignment with the divine and natural order that the very stones would shout out our arrival, is to enter our highest, anointed selves. And what New Testament tradition describes as Jesus' resurrection and return to the Father represents for us the possibility of a return to God by whatever name we choose to call it: the Higher Self, Brahman, the ground of Being.

This is heady stuff, I know. For most of us a mystical experience consists of finding a parking space with time left on the meter. For much of my life I've lived contentedly by a few simple rules: don't track mud in the house, take care of your own, help others, do as little harm as you can, change your oil every 3,000 miles. But maybe enlightenment is simpler than we think. I've been told that religion boils down to two beliefs: first, that there is something of ultimate significance in the universe; second, that there is a way of being connected to it. Each of the world's religions offers a distinct way of connecting, and each of us must find his or her own way in to ultimate significance. Prayer, meditation, and selfless service are all honored methods. The Buddhist monk Thich Nhat Hanh has taught me that, if done right, washing dishes can serve as well.

We also touch the Divine through our experience of nature, and in spring we celebrate the divine power of rebirth and renewal. Already the phoebes, after a journey unimaginable to me, have returned to their nest under the eaves outside my bedroom window. Their presence renews my faith in the world's extraordinary competence, its talent for winning against long odds. I breathe in the odor of wet earth and pines as though my sense of smell were being restored to me. All about us roots grip down and awaken. Sprouts nudge toward light and air. Everywhere the earth staggers to life.

And yet the example of Jesus, and the experience of mud season, also remind me of a harsher truth: to be reborn, we first must die. The way to Jerusalem lies through mud. Dying, like mud, can take many forms, but every death, in the sense I mean, is a letting go. We let go of ambition, of pride, of ego. We let go of relationships, of perfect health, of loved ones who go before us to their own deaths. We let go of insisting that the world be a certain way. Letting go of any of these things can seem the failure of every design, the loss of every cherished hope. But in letting them go, we may also let go fear, let go our white-knuckled grip on a life that never seems to meet our expectations, let go our anguished hold on smaller selves our spirits have outgrown. We may feel at times that we have let go of life itself, only to find ourselves in a new one, freer, roomier, more joyful than we could have imagined. We need not believe that Jesus rose bodily from the dead to grasp the spiritual significance of such a resurrection. In one of the ancient Gnostic gospels discovered at Nag Hammadi, an early Christian ridicules those who take the resurrection literally, saying instead that they must "receive the resurrection while they live." Another second century gnostic writer asks, "Why do you not examine your own self, and see that you have arisen?" (from Elaine Pagels, *The Gnostic Gospels*).

For much of my life I've been like the man in one of Rumi's poems, asleep indoors when a friend calls him out, saying that the mystics are gathering in the street. The sleeping man offers the excuse that he's sick, but his friend says: "I don't care if you're dead! Jesus is here, and he wants to resurrect somebody!" In my case it took more than a friend's shouting from the doorway to get me out of bed and into the street. It took the combined wisdom of several Harvard-trained neurologists to make me see that I needed to get up.

Before my illness I, like everyone, had always spent much of my time in the mud, only I didn't know to value it. Mud seemed only to block my way. I had spent my life in pursuit of knowledge and happiness, only to find out that both were overrated. For what is knowledge without faith, and what is happiness without sorrow? The path to resurrection lies through the mud because only through pain and sorrow do we grasp the necessary truth offered in the 90th psalm, rendered so beautifully by Stephen Mitchell:

> You return our bodies to the dust
> and snuff out our lives like a candleflame.
> You hurry us away; we vanish
> as suddenly as the grass:
> in the morning it shoots up and flourishes,
> in the evening it wilts and dies.
> For our life dissolves like a vision
> and fades into air like a cloud.

In the time it has taken me to write this essay, we in our part of New Hampshire have gone through an early thaw with bare ground showing on the southern slopes of the fields, through a week of single-digit temperatures, through another week of thaw and mud, through a blizzard that buried our hopes beneath a foot of snow, through a stretch of freakish 70 degree days in which snow vanished by the hour, and at last to gray days of cold rain. All this has reminded me of two things: the path to resurrection will be unpredictable, and we will have a hard time choosing the right footwear. Lately my daughter and I have come to an understanding. She wears her winter boots to school, but upon her return I meet her at the bus with her springtime rubber ones. She sits on a snowbank to pull them on, and then we stomp home through the mud. "Mud is good exercise," she says, searching for mud of just the right consistency to suck one boot off her foot. My father taught me to leave the stones in the road, to be prepared for mud. And now my children are learning from their father something about walking through it. They, in return, show me what spirit can be brought to the exercise. All of us, young and old, soon and late, find our way to the mud, the season of our terrible and certain joy. Let us bring to it all the spirit we can muster.

8

Choosing the World

My family and I recently spent two weeks out West looking at big things: volcanoes, canyons, oceans, redwoods. Exhilarating as it is, beauty on such a scale wearies me. Such great gobs of creation to be stuffed through the visual cortex, wrestled into thoughts, hoisted into memory. I feel too small for the job, as though I've been asked to measure the Columbia River with a thimble.

After looking at big things, it's a relief to come back to New Hampshire at berry picking time to focus on small ones: raspberries first, then a feast of blue. But it's a funny thing: standing in a berry patch, pinching fruit gently between my fingertips, I feel smaller still. In fact, when I attend to the smallest things, when I hand myself over to moss or mushroom, berry or beetle, I myself shrink to vanishing. This isn't as bad as it sounds, however. In fact, it's the reason we do such things. Anyone who's spent time on her knees in a berry patch or flower bed comes to see this attention to small things as a form of prayer, a way of vanishing, for one sweet hour, into whatever crumb of creation we are privileged to take into our hands.

If you have a transcendentalist streak, then at these moments of heightened attention to the visible world, you feel

closer to the invisible one. You may feel, with Emerson, that
"the visible creation is the terminus or the circumference of
the invisible world." And if you feel, as I do, a yearning to be
closer to God, perhaps there's no better place to be than in a
berry patch. This berry lifted to my lips is a simple material
fact, but one made sweeter by the thought that "a Fact is the
end or last issue of spirit" (Emerson again). But like Emerson
I worry that if I see the blueberry only as the visible mark of
some greater, invisible reality, then no matter how sweet,
the berry becomes second rate, a step removed from what
really counts. In this view the poor, profane berry, whose
powdered blue I rub to glossy black, is at best a gateway to
the sacred world, at worst an illusion and fraud. In my fixa-
tion on berries, I become a prisoner in Plato's cave, enter-
tained by shadows. Emerson's geometry is telling: if the visible world is but the "circumference" of the invisible one,
then we're forever outside the sacred circle at whose center
God lies. Only in mystic vision, or death, do we enter in.

Though even in death we may be denied. According to
many religious traditions, including Christian ones, my attachment to the things of this world disqualifies me for the
next. The berry's sweetness is my undoing. In the Hindu
tradition, I can't be released from the cycle of birth, suffering, and death until I can see the berry's dusky blue as a part
of *maya*, the veil of illusion that separates me from ultimate
reality. The Buddhist view is much the same, though to the
Buddhists the veil hides not the face of God but the essential
emptiness out of which all things come and to which they
return. And we know too well that according to the sterner
Christian doctrines a life of worldly pleasure leads to an afterlife involving skewers and flames.

These days, of course, most of us don't believe that we
must choose between the world and God. Some of us have
simply set aside such concerns altogether, figuring that if you
have to spend any time in a cave, Plato's or otherwise, it

might as well be one with berries in it. Even if we do worry about an afterlife, we figure that one sunny, breezy summer afternoon on the blueberry ledges may be worth a day or two in purgatory, if not an eternity rotating in the great rotisserie down below. But many of us who still believe in some sort of God have made an even more radical change from traditional ways of thinking. In the terms theologians like to use, we've moved away from notions of a transcendent God and embraced the idea of an immanent one. That is, we've gone from a distant, invisible, and otherworldly God to a God that is present and working within us and within the visible world of our experience. As Christian theologian Teilhard de Chardin writes, "Christ, through his Incarnation, is internal to the world, rooted in the world, even in the very heart of the tiniest atom." Jesus scholar Marcus Borg speaks for a lot of contemporary believers when he says that it's time to stop believing in God as a "supernatural being 'out there'," and time to start "being in relationship with a sacred reality 'right here'." In this view, the berry held between my fingertips is not the sign of some invisible, sacred world but a piece of sacredness itself. To taste its sweetness is to taste the Divine. This way, we can have our blueberry pie and eat it, too. We can choose the world, and in so doing choose God.

But I'm afraid I have made choosing God sound too easy. Who wouldn't choose a world of New Hampshire berry patches in July? But we all know that to embrace the world fully means choosing more than sunlit fields and berries and views of the White Mountains.

When I began writing this essay, men with chainsaws and a bulldozer were felling trees on our property to open up more of our view of Red Hill. As exciting as this was, I somehow found it hard to fix my mind upon the idea of a transcendent deity with chainsaws snarling outside my cabin. But if God is immanent in the world, then God is immanent also in the chainsaw, or at least in the beings who would invent and use it. Choosing the world means choosing all of it: the tall maple and the severed stump. In my case it means choosing a world that includes both black raspberry ice cream cones and my weakening arms, which will soon be unable to raise the ice cream to my lips. In choosing the world we choose both pleasure and pain, joy and sorrow, health and illness, rapture and rue.

Epimetheus, the Greek god who fashioned humans out of mud, learns this when Zeus presents him with a beautiful bride named Pandora. In accepting her he brings pleasure, companionship, and love into his house. He also brings a curiously heavy box with instructions never to let it be opened. I remember being told this story as a child, how upset I was when Pandora, giving in to curiosity and desire, opens the box, releasing evil and death into the world. It was like the Red Sox losing in the ninth inning—we had come so close! It has taken me a long time to understand that—like the Red Sox losing—the ending is inevitable. The box has to be opened. When Epimetheus chooses Pandora he chooses the box, too, without knowing the full implications of his choice. Merely by desiring Pandora he has, in a sense, already opened the box. Pandora, like Eve, her counterpart in Hebrew scripture, brings the knowledge that good and evil are inseparable, a wisdom she bears within her woman's body, the site of a lived and familiar intimacy between pain and pleasure, blood and birth. The story is not about distinguishing between right desires and wrong ones, or choosing between righteousness and sin. Rather, it tells us that desire itself, regardless of its object, enmeshes us in a world more complex than we first imagined, a world in which death and pleasure enter our homes together.

No wonder so many refuse the world. We all know about the obvious refusals—alcoholism, drug addiction, violence—but even the best of us at times fail to embrace life fully. How easy it is, when the world is too much with us, to retreat to the sofa with a stiff drink and the remote control. But whether our evasions of the world take this or other forms, choosing the world, in the radical way I mean it, involves more than getting up off of the sofa, more than just keeping busy. For I want to choose the world in such a way that I am choosing God, too.

Sometimes it's our very busyness that gets in the way of such a choice. Too often we anesthetize ourselves by setting up our lists and ambitions and accomplishments as a shield between us and our true selves. We strap ourselves into our carefully constructed identities for fear of letting go into the pain and wonder that awaits just the other side of our precious reserve. In a culture that recognizes busyness as the mark of importance and worth, it's so easy to use our public identities—as professionals, as caretakers and volunteers, as overworked parents—to avoid all that's troubling, complex and mysterious in the world around us. When I was a young teacher and a student came to me with a problem, I too often retreated behind the mask of my hard-won professorial status. I wore tweed jackets and the grave expression of a man thinking deep thoughts. I was there to teach literature and write important books, I told myself, and didn't have time to help 18-year-olds adjust to living away from home. Behind my impatience and emotional stinginess was of course my own insecurity, my fear that by stepping outside the carefully policed enclosure of professional identity I would reveal too much of my own messy humanity, which would do no one any good. Friends who are doctors tell me the same thing: how easy it is, in the face of a patient's anguish and fear, to maintain a carefully practiced professional reserve as a defense against empathy. And yet, as we all know, the best physicians and teachers manage somehow to express their humanity at the same time as they exercise their professional skill. When former students write to me, I'm surprised by what they remember: books and ideas, yes, but also the smell of popcorn in my house, or the blues guitar I played once in the college coffeehouse, or a passing comment I made and quickly forgot but which helped them through a difficult time. Harried, overworked, and overwhelmed as we are, we often experience our students, patients, clients, colleagues, and children as difficult, irresponsible, rude, dull, or simply too numerous to keep track of. But if we mean to choose the world, we must see God in the people who come under our care. That is, we must see them as at bottom no different from ourselves. No matter our busyness, no matter our own or others' flaws, we need at some point to see every human being as a marvel, a berry held up in sunlight, worthy of wonder.

I don't mean to make it sound as though choosing the world is just a matter of being *nice*. Indeed, a more pernicious, because more subtle, refusal of our world comes when we retreat into our own goodness. Thomas Merton, the great scholar, writer, and monastic, is especially insightful on this point. To him, choosing the world in such a way that we also choose God isn't merely a question of obeying the rules and avoiding sin. In fact, in Merton's more challenging view, it's often our assurance of our own goodness that blocks our approach to the Divine. Merton, a Catholic, writes that the genius of Protestantism in its original, radical form was its focus not on converting the wicked but on "a much more difficult and problematic conversion, that of the pious and the good." Protestant religion gets into trouble, Merton says, when, "forgetting the seriousness of the need to convert the good, [it] bogs down in the satisfied complacency of a rather superficial and suburban goodness—the folksy togetherness, the hand-shaking fellowship, the garrulous witness of moral platitudes. (In this of course Protestants are often outdistanced by the more complex and sometimes more vulgar inanities of the 'good Catholic')." How often do we substitute perfunctory goodness for a genuine, loving engagement with others? I think of how easily I write a check to help the homeless, and of how hard it is for me to look a homeless person in the eye. I'm reminded of a Peanuts cartoon in which the character Linus says, "I love humanity. It's people I can't stand."

Reacting against both the busyness of our materialistic culture and the superficial goodness of religion as it can be practiced in our churches, many people these days are searching for spirituality in new places. Too often, however, New Age and other spiritual practices tempt us with cheap transcendence. Handed a mantra or mandala or medicine wheel, we do a swift end run past pain and loss, turn the corner on mystery and darkness, and sprint downfield toward bliss. I'm as guilty in this department as anyone. Searching for both spiritual and physical healing in the face of my Lou Gehrig's disease, I've done my share of chanting and drumming; people have massaged my energy field and consorted with celestial beings on my behalf. I have on my desk a packet containing the ashes of the burnt hair of some saintly man living in India. A kind and intelligent woman gave me this after a sermon I delivered in her church. Apparently I'm supposed to eat the ashes or drink them in tea, and I might just do it. I can't say what good all these things have done me, other than provide some hours of distraction from the rigors of my imperfect life. Some days it's simply easier to contemplate my chakras than to contemplate the mystery of my failing flesh—just as sometimes it's easier to embrace a realm of pure light than a world containing cranky children and a sink full of dirty dishes.

To choose the world, then, doesn't mean to evade it through busyness, or to rest in easy moral certainties, or to imagine that surrendering to God's will is something like surrendering to a hammock on a Sunday afternoon.

But then how *do* we choose the world, and on what terms?

We begin by recognizing that the world is not separate from ourselves. Honoring the world in all its complexity, all its light and shadow, means honoring myself most fully, and recognizing that I and the world have a common source. When I hold the berry in my hand, and when in contemplation of that bit of sacredness I begin to vanish, there's a sense in which the berry, too, vanishes, as though we were but two drops returned to the well of being. To see the world in this way, as Thomas Merton writes, "means not the rejection of a reality, but the unmasking of an illusion. The world as pure object is something that is not there. It is not a reality outside us for which we exist. . . . We and our world interpenetrate." Rather than seeing the visible world as the limit or circumference of the invisible one, then, at such moments in the berry patch we no longer see a difference between visible and invisible, matter and spirit. These distinctions simply disappear. Emerson himself, in pulling back from strict transcendentalism, arrived at this view eventually. Using a striking metaphor, he writes: "Nature is so pervaded with human life, that there is something of humanity in all, and in every particular. . . . Therefore spirit, that is, the Supreme Being, does not build up nature around us, but puts it forth through us, as the life of the tree puts forth new branches and leaves through the pores of the old."

In other words, the world we choose hasn't been imposed on us from without, but comes into being *through* us. In every moment we collaborate in the ongoing work of creation, including the creation of ourselves. For Joan Chittister, the Benedictine monastic, "we work because the world is unfinished and it is ours to develop." Work, therefore, become a sacred responsibility, and choosing the world means choosing what we ourselves have made. As Merton writes, "It is only in assuming full responsibility for our world, for our lives and for ourselves that we can be said to live really for God." To be responsible is to be responsive, to respond. All these words have their root in the Latin *spondeo*, which means "to promise." To re-spond is not to promise for the first time, but to promise again, not to begin a relationship, but to renew one.

One evening this spring, I sat at the dinner table with my children, Amelia and Aaron, ages 7 and almost 9. The first flies were hatching and, drawn to the light of the house, gathering on the window pane near us. Struck with a sudden enthusiasm, the kids got pencils and paper and began to draw. Ignoring the moths and more obvious bugs, they chose as their subject a tiny white-winged fly, perhaps two millimeters wide, so small you wouldn't have noticed it unless you were looking hard.

Now my son, the older of the two, had had some practice at such things, but my daughter's drawings had so far been limited in subject to standard if charming flowers and rainbows and butterflies and little brown-haired girls. She had never tried drawing a tiny white fly, or in fact to draw anything at all that was actually before her in the world rather than summoned from her imagination. And sure enough, her first sketch of the fly looked suspiciously like those brightly colored butterflies that had flown beneath so many smiling suns in the works that until then made up her principal *oeuvre*. When I suggested she go back and look more closely at the fly's antennas, you could see the flash of recognition in her face. She got up from the table and crouched by the window. She looked, she looked again, she pressed her nose to the glass, she returned to the table. Erasing what she had drawn before, she first got the antennas right, then went back to the window to study the legs. Each time she came back to the table, her paper got more smudged with erasures, but she managed to get the right number of legs in the right places and bent at the correct angles, then to tackle the wings, the body, the head.

Our responsibilities to the world are many and complex, yet they seem to begin here, in this simple yet arduous act of seeing the world and responding—renewing our promise—

to it. I sometimes imagine that if the creator of the universe wanted to take another shot at communicating what was most important, she might replace all of sacred scripture with the words "Pay Attention!" To choose the world means first of all to see it clearly, to shed fantasy and habit, to look, and look again, to let ourselves be broken open by its intricacy and its mystery. It's fitting that one source for the word *religion* is a group of words meaning "to read again," for we must return to the book of the world for a closer reading. Only when we have read and reread with open mind and heart can we fruitfully carry on God's work. Then, picking up our pencils, we continue the world's unfinished text.

Again I may have made all this sound too easy, as though looking closely at bugs and berries were all that were required for our enlightenment. The problem is that seeing is never plain. The woman who has just found a new lover gazes out her kitchen window at the overgrown lawn and sees there luxuriance, a wild and delicious excess. The man who has just lost his job looks out the same window at the same lawn and sees there more evidence of his decline. There is always something *behind* our seeing, something prior to it. Even the so-called "objective" standpoint of the scientist, however valuable and important, is not an absolute frame of reference but rather grows out of a particular set of interests and concerns. Thus the question arises: if we must see the world clearly in order to choose it, what world must we see?

This question has long been the province of various ologies—epistemology, phenomenology, ontology—that have kept generations of philosophy professors busy. But the basic issues at stake are easy enough to grasp. Choosing the world in the way I mean it takes something in addition to scientific seeing, something that I'll call "mystical seeing." Now, I know that in a culture where scientific, rational and secular values dominate, the word "mystical" has at best come to stand for all that is uselessly poetic and obscure, and at worst has become a synonym for mistaken, fuzzy headed, or just plain wacko. But mystical experience isn't all that unusual. Most of us have found that a line of poetry or scripture, a passage of music, the turning of a leaf in sunlight, or the sight of a child splashing in a stream can suddenly become a doorway through which, as William James writes, "the mystery of fact, the wildness and the pang of life, steals into our hearts and thrills them." Each of the world religions has a mystical tradition wherein such experiences are cultivated and understood within the context of a person's normal spiritual development. We have in large part lost touch with these traditions, and these days most people encounter them only in distorted, New Age forms that can make them seem at odds with reason and the demands of everyday life. That's a pity, for as a "rational mystic" I've found that by integrating my mystical side with my scientific one I'm best able, every day, to renew my promise to a world vitally charged with meaning. I would have us learn to see as both scientists and mystics, for we need both kinds of vision for the fullest possible apprehension of life.

I know a man who gained an international reputation as a botanical illustrator, selling his work regularly to *National Geographic* and other publications. For years he drew plants and insects not only with scientific accuracy but great artistic beauty. And yet, for all his practiced attention to small things, for all his reading and re-reading of the book of the world, he did not see his art as a spiritual activity. Then, after spending time among Native Americans in the Southwest, he learned to see in a new way. The world had become sacred to him. The shift to mystic seeing transformed his art—along with the rest of his life. He now does relatively little illustration work, instead making paintings that he considers a form of prayer. Explaining this to me one day in his studio, he showed me a piece that dramatized this shift in vision. The painting depicted a monarch butterfly and a single leaf of a begonia, each rendered in the exquisite detail and brilliant pigment of his former "scientific" work. In this painting, however, the butterfly and leaf float over a formless charcoal sky through which drifts a full moon. Thus the scientific vision emerges from the mystical one, with order and precision set against a background of chaos and mystery.

Scientific seeing, for good reasons, seeks to fix the world like a bug pinned to a tray, wants to make it fully *present* to our rational understanding. Mystical seeing, on the other hand, discovers both presence and absence equally. When I hold the berry in my hand, when I surrender myself wholly to its presence, I know I'm in the presence of the Divine. But at the same time, I come to know the berry as a mystery beyond my comprehension, and I come to know God as that which is essentially unknowable. Mystical seeing always involves this paradox, and thus can be as harrowing as it is uplifting. To approach God is to know the infinite distance between God and us; to know God is to enter what one medieval mystic called "the cloud of unknowing." Each moment of light and clarity brings darkness and confusion. I possess all knowledge, all wisdom, all joy, and at the same moment I'm empty and cast down, groveling with Job before the voice out of the whirlwind. Mystical seeing exhalts us at the same time as it knocks us out of our complacency, our confidence, our righteousness. (That's why true mystics have so often been labeled troublemakers and heretics: they refuse the comforts of orthodoxy.) To live in the world opened up by this larger perspective requires what Keats called "negative capability," the poet's ability to be "in uncertainties, mysteries, doubts, without any irritable reaching after fact and reason." The mystic, like the poet, like all of us who seek the fullest apprehension of life, must leave the settled world of the known to dwell in the wilderness of mystery.

But you can choose the world without writing poetry or living in a desert cave. You need no equipment other than the human heart. The anonymous medieval mystic who wrote *The Cloud of Unknowing* tells us that "all rational beings possess two faculties, the power of knowing and the power of loving. To the first, to the intellect, God who made them is forever unknowable, but to the second, to love, he is completely knowable, and that by every separate individual." We must see the world as scientists, but first as lovers. Growing up in a world fearful of mystery, we've fallen out of the habit, and must relearn it. We must love the world with a child's love for its parents, a love immediate and unreserved, no matter that the world gives us both blueberries and the black flies that torment us as we pick them. We must love the world with a love of a mother or father for her or his two-year-old child, the one with the scabby knees and runny nose and the lungs of a future opera singer running toward us now with whatever gob of creation—wasp nest or worm or wisteria—it has clutched in its gleeful fist. We must love the world as new lovers do one another, as if to be in the beloved's presence is to walk through a world made newly luminous, finding that every ordinary gesture—the way he drops his car keys on the table, the way she raises a cup to her lips—is holy and part of a sacred dance. Mystic vision is a lover's vision, and despite the pain love brings, to see the world through a lover's eyes is already to have chosen it.

Our first act upon entering the world is to draw breath, to take some of its substance into ourselves. And with our first exhalation we give something of ourselves back to the world. The world moves through us as we move through the world, each breath a response, a renewal of that original promise. To choose the world is to return to where we began, to follow love to its source, to rest in that ground of our being that has no beginning and no ending. Moved by love of the world, we venture all to enter the sacred circle, to cross the threshold of the invisible, to draw closer to God. When at last we find ourselves there, inside the world's holy heart, we discover we have been there all along. Born of the world, we give birth to the world in every moment. Beloved of the world, we are every moment in its embrace. Choosing the world, we discover in the end that the world has already chosen us.

9

WINTER MIND

One must have a mind of winter
To regard the frost and the boughs
Of the pine-trees crusted with snow;

And have been cold a long time
To behold the junipers shagged with ice,
The spruces rough in the distant glitter

Of the January sun; and not to think
Of any misery in the sound of the wind

from "The Snow Man," Wallace Stevens

I have on my office door these words from an accomplished
Indian yogi: "Before speaking, consider whether it is an
improvement upon silence." The man who wrote them once
went 19 years without speaking, setting a standard I can't hope
to meet. Yet his words remind me that when we do speak, we
must speak truth. Even more important, because truth so often eludes us, we must speak in kindness. In fact, we might
amend the yogi's saying to read, "Before speaking, consider
whether you speak out of love." If we could learn always to

speak out of love, we could change everything, and maybe I should end this essay right here. But I have more to say about silence, about how we might bring silence into our lives and thereby make both our speaking and our doing more fruitful. I'm speaking of that silence both ordinary and profound, the fundamental silence out of which words come and to which they return. The word *infant* means "without speech," and as infants we're allowed a few months of wordless union with our mothers. Our first cries express our desire to be returned to our mother's breast, and as soon as we are weaned from that breast, we start talking. We talk our lives away, unaware that no amount of speech will get us back to where we really want to be. The fall into language is our expulsion from the garden, our fall into that separateness by which we gain a self, a speaking self whose words can do little more than mark the absence of all they signify. Only death shuts us up. From silence we come, and unto silence we will return. In the meantime, we talk. In a *New Yorker* cartoon, a gravestone reads: "Born 1932. Yada yada yada. Died 1995."

But we don't have to die to experience silence. We all have memories of important silences in our lives. I recall, from my New Hampshire youth, lying in a hayloft watching dust dance in a shaft of sunlight, and I recall looking down the front of Arlene Colebrook's dress in the snack booth at the Old Home Week penny sale, both occasions of wordless awe. At such moments we don't choose silence, but *fall* silent. Silence, like love, is not something we reason our way into. And once we are in it, we recognize that it has been there all along. It's there like the background noise of the universe, that uniform hiss astronomers find when they point their radio telescopes at the space between stars, the remnant of the Big Bang, the residual wind of our origin.

But let me speak of another wind, this one nearer home. I want to tell you about the sound of winter wind through a New Hampshire forest. Some of you have heard the sound I mean, though it's heard only in great stretches of northern woods, far from freeways and flight paths, and if you haven't been to such a place lately, you will have to work to remember it. It's the sound a whole forest makes, unlocatable and everywhere, near and far, intimate and impossibly remote. I do not mean a storm wind, full of high drama, but the gentle, subtle voice of a forest as it speaks of winter peace and winter desolation.

The forest where we live is mixed hardwoods and conifers: maple, oak, beech, and birch; white pine, spruce, and hemlock. Two mountain ridges lie between me and the interstate highway twenty miles off, and with no sizable town in earshot, I can hear the sound such a forest makes when gently dithered by winter air. Leaves are down, of course, so it's the pines that matter most. They stand tallest and catch the wind. Theirs is a finely sifted sound, a soft hiss through unnumbered needles. Stand by one as it takes the air, and you'll know how God breathes. Hear the accumulated sound of such trees coming at you over the miles, and you hear something like the breath of Being itself, the very sigh of our becoming and passing away. The ground must be covered in snow to keep the sound pure, free of shrub turbulence and dead leaf scuttle. And there's more: hardwoods, their bare branches stiffened, provide an undertone, low and harder edged, the barely audible drag of sticks through cold air. And last, close by: the rattle of dead beech leaves still clinging to their boughs.

Most often the sound steals up on me, as I pause between house and barn, or while I'm crunching down the dirt road to meet the children's school bus or opening the door at night to call the dog. I hear this wind in its purest form only a handful of times each winter, yet when I do I imagine it has been there always, back of everything else I thought I was doing with my life. Whenever I hear it, I think: surely this is the sound I heard as I was born, the sound I will hear as I die.

But perhaps I'm getting too serious here. Winter does

take us to extremes. John Donne, in a winter solstice poem written over three centuries ago, moans that "the whole world's sap is sunk." And so it is: maples stand brittle in the cold wind, their fluids drained to the roots. The earth cools, life hides in holes. Winter locks us in our solid states, flinty and frozen. My world goes nearly inorganic. The air's dryer, the stars give a harder glint. There's a purity to it all, of course. A cleanliness. And at the brink of lifelessness our taste for life grows keen. Wallace Stevens understood this when he wrote, "It is here, in this bad, that we reach / The last purity of the knowledge of good."

Whenever I read the poem in which these lines appear (Stevens' "No Possum, No Sop, No Taters"), I recall boyhood nights when I went sledding by moonlight. This went best when several feet of snow had been followed by rain and then a freeze, forming an icy crust that was dangerously fast and just hard enough to bear the weight of children and dogs. Grownups would punch through up to their thighs, so that they couldn't follow us when after dinner we trooped out into a neighbor's field glowing with moonlight. Stevens had it right: "Snow sparkles like eyesight falling to earth, / Like seeing fallen brightly away." Walking out to the top of the sloping field, my younger brother and I with the neighbor's kids, we filled the night with our noise: boastful chatter, the dull booming of our molded plastic sleds held and struck like gongs. But there came a moment at the top of the field when we fell silent, looking down over that creamy slope toward the dark woods waiting at the bottom. In silence we lined up our sleds, lay flat on our bellies, noses just inches above the snow. It was a sobering business, and that was how we wanted it. For me then—twelve or fourteen years old—the essence of good sledding was fear. Speed mattered, and anything that amplified the sense of speed was welcome. Hence darkness, cold, the absence of grownups, the waiting woods. Like all adolescent boys, we were in love with our own annihilation.

There was no end to those woods, we knew. They sunk into swamp, rose over hills, and in our minds swept on forever into Canada and the frozen north. Our goal was to plunge into them, to be swallowed up, and then to return victorious. The key was not to bail out too soon and so be cheated of glory. We knew that on this icy crust, on sleds of hard plastic, we would quickly reach a terminal velocity of several hundred miles an hour. We knew, too, that our glossy nylon parkas had a coefficient of friction only slightly higher than that of plastic, so that when we did bail out, we would continue sliding on our backs, watching the wall of the woods rise over us like a dark wave until we tore through the brambles at the field's edge, broke through alder and willow saplings, and carried on to keep our final appointment with a stone wall topped with barbed wire. *This* was good sledding.

When the run was over, and I lay bruised and torn and unbearably happy, the silence would fall. And that's when I would hear it: the winter wind, breathing from the miles of forest at whose edge I lay, that chill spirit mingling with my own breath rising in plumes toward the brilliant moon, the cold stars. I would lie there a long time, feeling my back cool, my whole body cool toward the temperature of snow, listening to that wind that was hardly a wind, that subtle non-sound. At such times I would know what Stevens wants us to know in another of his poems, "The Snowman": "One must have a mind of winter . . . / And have been cold a long time . . . not to think / Of any misery in the sound of the wind." To be of winter mind is to be so empty of preconception as to hear without judgment and thus to hear in that wind neither misery nor happiness. Such a "listener, who listens in the snow," beholds the world without delusion or projection, seeing "nothing that is not there." To have a mind of winter requires, however, that the listener be "nothing himself". Lying in the snow, I let my body cool, my breath slow, my mind empty of thoughts. The winter mind, knowing its own emptiness, beholds "nothing that is not there" but also, as its final achievement, "the nothing that is." At this moment of merging, one emptiness beholds another emptiness not different from itself. All separateness falls away, and I am one with snow and stars, rooted as pine, imperturbable as stone. This may seem quite an accomplishment for a boy on a plastic sled, but adolescents are natural mystics. I suspect that most of us can recall such moments from the years when the snow's crust still bore our weight. In childhood we enter naturally those realms of spirit that as adults we touch only through conscious effort and practice. The world itself is the child's cathedral, and so it may be for us adults, if we can relearn our childlike openness to it.

John Tarrant's wonderful book, *The Light Inside the Dark*, lay on my desk as I was writing this. Seeing it, and sounding out the title, my seven-year-old daughter asked, "How can there be light inside the dark?" It took her half a second to answer her own question: "Oh, yes, the moon."

Which returns me to that dreamy adolescent lying at the edge of a moonlit field, for I think I can learn something more from him. This essay, like good sledding, begins with silence and moonlight and goes down the slippery slope toward emptiness. "Emptiness"—the usual translation for the Sanskrit term *sunyata*—occupies a central place in Buddhist thought. From the Prajnaparamita, or Heart Sutra (one of Buddhism's central texts), we learn that "emptiness is no other than form; form is no other than emptiness." Here, as in so many sacred texts, paradoxical language gestures toward something that cannot be grasped by intellect alone. Just as silence is the necessary condition or ground of speech, emptiness is not negation but pure possibility, the condition or ground of being. And as with the silence I spoke of earlier, to become aware of it is to know that it's been there all along. As John Tarrant writes: "The emptiness is the host of which we are every moment the guest. . . . The empty realm is not a place we may live in, but if we want freedom, we must pass through it. It is the gate of spiritual initiation, the destination to which our sincerity, our foolishness, our suffering, our meditation and prayer have led us."

And like good sledding, the slide toward emptiness can be scary. Emptiness sounds too much like nothingness, and our work in this world is all about its opposite, somethingness. We're told to make something of ourselves; we want to be somebody. These are the callings and warnings of ego, and they're not all bad: in responding to them we create something not only for ourselves but for our children and for our communities. We have good reasons to dread nothingness and to spend our lives avoiding it.

In most western philosophical traditions nothingness means loss, negation, death, the void. But the Buddhists see things differently. In a cartoon I saw once, it's the Dalai Lama's birthday, and he's opening a gift-wrapped box, which turns out to be empty. Looking into it, the Dalai Lama says: "Nothing. Just what I've always wanted!"

You can think of this essay as offering the gift of an empty box, but you shouldn't think of me as having offered it. I merely point out that the gift has already been offered, is offered to you at every moment, is in fact all around you and within you, available as breath. All that remains is for you to accept it. That's both easier and harder than it sounds. Emptiness, like silence, like love, is not something we choose, not something we reason our way into, but rather something into which we fall, something in which we *find ourselves*. The fall into emptiness, into silence, has the nature of an accident. And though we can't choose our accidents, we can learn to make ourselves accident prone. We can point our sleds downhill. There's a Sanskrit word, *sthita*, which means "standing firm," or "taking a position." In Hindu painting and statuary, the gods and goddesses practice *sthita* by taking physical postures emblematic of their particular spiritual natures. While we cannot choose emptiness, we can choose to practice *sthita*, and thereby make ourselves available for the fall into emptiness, which always comes as a grace. There are many ways to practice *sthita:* you can meditate, attend religious services, practice Bach études. What matters is that you find some way to point your sled downhill. You don't know where you'll land—*sthita* is an act of faith—but you must be willing to take the ride.

Now, on its face, preparing to hurtle down-slope on a plastic sled would seem to have little to do with *sthita*, or "standing firm." But I mean to suggest a paradox at the heart of this book. Falling, in the way I mean it, means finding a stillness in the midst of life's calamitous downhill rush. And in sitting silently, we prepare ourselves to fall. Silence, in fact, lies at the heart of spiritual practice in many of the world's religions. In the most common form of Buddhist meditation, one sits silently, often for long periods, continually returning the awareness to the breath, to this wind of our origin and of our passing away. Our word "spirit" comes from the Latin *spiritus*, or "breath"; in returning to the breath, we return to spirit, we hear the winter wind, we allow ourselves to cool into winter mind, we prepare for the fall into emptiness. And in touching emptiness we touch the source, the spring, the creative power out of which the universe flows at every moment. That source has many names, but I call it "God."

Americans seem to think Asian religions have a lock on emptiness, just as in the '70s we thought that only the Japanese could make quality automobiles. I'm struck, though, by how much the Buddhist tradition I have been describing has in common with Christian mysticism and the long tradition of the *via negativa*, which emphasizes God's essential unknowability. Meister Eckhart, the medieval Christian mystic, who belongs to this tradition, tells us quite bluntly that "people should stand empty." He advocates a radical letting go, not only of material possessions but of intellectual and spiritual ones as well. "Blessed are the poor in spirit," and for Eckhart the truly poor in spirit let go of all knowledge, including the knowledge of God; they let go of all will, even the will to do the will of God. As Matthew Fox comments, "It is this radical letting go of willing, of knowing, and of having that allows God to enter." Many who reject traditional Christianity find Buddhism attractive because it seems like a way to have religion without having God. But Eckhart's God is far from the bearded old man in the clouds. In fact, Eckhart does not believe in a personal deity of any description, and at his most radical, the line between his notion of God and the Buddhist conception of ultimate reality vanishes. He writes: "The masters say that God is a being, an intelligent being, and that he knows all things. We say, however: God is neither being nor intelligent nor does he know this or that. Thus God is free of all things, and therefore he is all things." Eckhart also says provocatively: "I pray God to rid me of God." By this he expresses his desire to be rid of any notion of a God that stands separate and apart from himself. Merely to utter the name of God, or to say that God "enters in," is to "preserve distinction," to continue to place ourselves apart from God. In our moments of highest realization we stand so empty as to have merged with our source, and in that state no words are necessary. We have returned to the great silence from which we came.

On a recent night I found I couldn't sleep, so some time after midnight I went to my study to read Meister Eckhart's sermons. As profound as this experience was, after an hour or so I set the book aside and picked up the L.L. Bean catalog. Nothingness is great, I thought, but that's a really nice sweater. We never leave our humanness behind, and we aren't supposed to. It's not a matter of choosing between spirit and world. Instead, we must let the things of this world become, as John Tarrant puts it, "stained through with spirit." Our current situation demands mystics who can balance their checkbooks, get the kids to school, and put food on the table. We are called not to sit in a cave, or even to lie at the edge of a moonlit field, but to see every object and every action against the luminous background of emptiness. In the midst of our working and doing we take our stand, we open ourselves to emptiness, as John Tarrant writes, "bringing the great background near, so that whatever we do, rising in the quiet, has force and beauty." Coming out of silence each word gains substance; coming out of emptiness each action grows distinct. In practicing *sthita*, in taking our stand, we find ourselves free, regardless of our circumstances, to speak in kindness and act for the good.

These days, my own relationship with silence grows more intimate. With Lou Gehrig's disease I face the loss of my ability to speak, just as I am now losing my ability to walk. Already my speech slows, my tongue grows unwieldy. Before hefting another syllable across my palate I consider more seriously whether it will improve upon silence. Because I'm too dense to get the message any other way, and despite my years of meditation, the fates are instructing me quite literally in the art of sitting down and shutting up. I'm being shown what is essential. But my situation only dramatizes the choice we all face. Whatever our personal circumstances, we can resist our fate and continue to suffer, or we can open ourselves to the fall into emptiness. We can choose to point our sleds downhill. The dark woods are waiting, but also the moon.

A friend recently forwarded me this poem, e-mailed to him from Japan:

> if you have time to chatter, read books.
> if you have time to read, walk to mountain, desert, ocean.
> if you have time to walk, sing songs and dance.
> if you have time to dance, sit quietly you Happy Lucky Idiot.

As a season of the spirit , winter can seize us any time of year. When it does, may we open ourselves to emptiness, that we may know the blessings of winter mind. May we come to know, in this bad, the last purity of the knowledge of good. May we come to know what happy, lucky idiots we are.

I wish you good sledding.

10

THE ART OF DOING NOTHING

I once knew a woman from Louisiana who fell in love with a man from New England. One summer, they planted a garden together. Now, for the woman a garden was a lush and fragrant place with big drowsy-scented blooms and dark foliage creeping and climbing and drooping and maybe some space for hot chili peppers and Chinese eggplants. The New England man planted potatoes and turnips, carrots and cabbage. It took them some time to come to terms with their differences. For her the garden meant luxury and pleasure. For him it meant survival.

The man or woman who measures well-being by the size of the woodpile and the quantity of onions stashed in the cellar may find the art of doing nothing impossible to master. But it's not just New Englanders who suffer from the compulsion to keep busy. Americans in general cannot rest from doing and acquiring, as though some winter of the spirit, if not of climate, were always just around the corner. Keeping busy for us is not just a practical matter but an ethical one. We equate doing nothing with idleness, and we all know idle hands do the devil's work. The French, who have added to the Ten Commandments an eleventh—thou shalt take six weeks of vacation every summer—have an easier time with leisure than we do.

Many of us do vacations badly, and so in summer we find ourselves in trouble. We may look forward to vacation all year, but when the time arrives, we grow anxious. Will I have enough to do, we ask. Or will I be doing the *right* things? Can I stand spending that much time with my family? Can I stand spending that much time with myself? Our habits of busyness cannot easily be switched off, and many of us concoct vacations that seem suspiciously like work. We propel ourselves over land and water at life-threatening speeds, we trudge up and down mountains until we're too tired to speak, we succumb to fits of power gardening. Even when we tune up the lawn chairs and settle in for some serious idleness, we find it hard to leave behind our competitive instincts. Last summer, I enjoyed sitting in the meadow in the early morning to take the air and watch the birds and insects do their work. I counted myself lucky. But when I got a post card from a friend who had just defended his family against a grizzly bear while hiking in Montana, I felt somehow outdone. Now that's a vacation, I thought.

Some of us can't stand to leave off work at all. My wife and I have both been blessed with finding work we loved, and so we suffered through the third week of our honeymoon, during which it became clear to us that *two* weeks of blissful leisure was about as much as we could take. Wanting to be back home working, we instead had to endure the torment of a week's hiking in the Swiss Alps, ogling glaciers, sleeping in abandoned sheep barns, and dancing to accordion music in rustic mountain huts. Eventually we solved our problem by moving to this small New Hampshire town, a place of mountains and lakes and mosquitoes where you can pretend you're on vacation while working constantly.

We Americans get little credit for doing nothing, so it's

no wonder we're not very good at it. We speak of the Protestant work ethic, which derives from that peculiar Calvinist pathology that sees our good works as signs of our election to the ranks of the saved. According to that old doctrine (can you say "predestinarianism"?), each of us was given the big thumbs up or thumbs down way back before Adam bit into that first juicy macintosh, each quivering soul paraded before a judging God in a place I always imagined as looking like the council of Odin in the Thor comic books I kept in the hayloft of our barn and would read on those long, lazy prelapsarian boyhood summer afternoons when I still knew the blessings of idleness and had not yet fallen into the obsession with work and accomplishment that seems to infect all who land upon this mortal shore.

But if Calvinism is the bug that infects us, it's a remarkably adaptable germ, having flourished in the blood of my own forebears, who were Irish and German Catholics and European Jews, and finding hosts among Mexicans, Guatemalans, Koreans, Egyptians, Palestinians, Indonesians, Cambodians, and other decidedly non-Protestant immigrants whose work ethic enriches our nation every day. And it has flourished despite its own illogic: if our fates have already been decided in advance, if each of us has already been booked into either the boiler room or the penthouse suite at the Afterlife Hotel, then why worry about proving ourselves in this life? But human behavior isn't driven by logic, and despite its repudiation by most religious thinkers today, Calvinism continues to tap a deep current of the human psyche. We work in the hopeful if deluded belief that we can control our fates, in this world or the next. Our work denies our doom.

Sometimes, of course, our busyness has less to do with theology or dark compulsion than with simple necessity. The world needs our activity, our doing and our care. There are children to be fed, students to be taught, houses to be built, gardens to be tended. There is too much injustice, too much need, too many openings for love, to justify our sitting idle. And on my hopeful days, I like to think also that we work for sheer love of goodness and beauty.

But we all know something's wrong when our working gets in the way of our living, when our doing leaves us disconnected from others and ourselves. There are two kinds of busyness, one of quantity and one of quality. With the first kind of busyness we take on so many worthwhile tasks that it begins to seem like a kind of neurosis. Did I really need to volunteer again for the balloon inflation committee for the annual Zucchini Festival parade? Did I really need to make that second trip to the store for the box of Eggo waffles when I could just have said, "Let them eat toast"? Each day, we want to do what is most important, but not knowing what that one task might be, we take on 12 or 50, like the student taking an exam who writes down every possible answer, hoping that one of them will be right. At times we glimpse the difficult truth in these lines from the *Tao Te Ching*:

> A truly good man does nothing,
> Yet leaves nothing undone.
> A foolish man is always doing,
> Yet much remains to be done.

But what can that mean? How can a truly good man do nothing? These questions bring us to the second kind of busyness, which isn't as much about doing a lot as it is about having a busy mind. The art of doing nothing involves more than sitting still. These days as walking gets more difficult, I'm getting lots of practice sitting still, and I'm learning the difference between that and doing nothing. As I said, last summer, I tried to spend part of each morning in my wheelchair looking out across the lawn, over the stone wall and across acres of meadow to where Red Hill rises over the forest. Swallows snatch bugs over the field, the phoebe tends her nest above the doorway, a breeze stirs about my ankles as somewhere in the forest an oven bird makes its ratchet-y commentary on the nature of time. Meanwhile I'm thinking about the pile of loam in my yard that somebody has got to do something with; I'm thinking that if so and so doesn't show up with his tractor pretty soon and start mowing, that field is going to go entirely to goldenrod; I'm thinking of screens to be put up and windows to be washed; I'm thinking that none of these things am I able to do myself. I'm thinking of the mountain of wood chips in my driveway, that I've got to find someone to spread the chips around the shrubs that have yet to be planted in front of the deck that I've got to get the carpenters to finish. And while I'm trying not to think about how I'm going to pay for all of this, I'm thinking of the culvert that's got to be put in the driveway and whether the plumber will ever get the bathtub fixtures to match the sink fixtures and whether we should return those towel rods to Home Depot, and get the chrome ones with the brass accents. I'm thinking I should check my email and that I'd better have the nozzles replaced on my color printer; I'm thinking that I don't know enough about Web page design and I'm wondering if my literary agent is ever going to do anything for me or should I dump him and find somebody else and then I'm thinking it's not the agent, it's me, and maybe I should give up writing and instead get serious about learning Sanskrit, and then I'm thinking my coffee has gone cold and I've managed to waste most of a morning staring at this dammed view again.

Why do we do this to ourselves? A mischievous meditation teacher once told a group of us not to worry about all this busyness inside our heads. "It's not such a big deal," he said. "After all, it's just a question of how we spend our time every second for the rest of our lives."

I think if we're honest with ourselves, we can agree that our busyness—whether of body or of mind—is often a distraction, a way of avoiding others, avoiding intimacy, avoiding ourselves. We keep busy to push back our fears, our lone-liness, our self-doubt, our questions about purposes and ends. We want to know we matter, we want to know our lives are worthwhile. And when we're not sure, we work that much harder, we worry that much more. In the face of our uncer-tainty, we keep busy. These days, the idea of original sin has grown unfashionable, but to me it seems as good a way as any of naming that deep feeling of unworthiness so many of us suffer, driving us to hurl a lifetime of work and worry into a pit that can never be filled. Unchecked, this impulse can drag us into bitterness, loneliness, depression, and despair.

What is it, then, that restores us to a better version of ourselves, that returns us to our firm sense of goodness—both our own and the world's? Perhaps it's a question of grace: a reflected sunset flares in the windows of a skyscraper, a sheet of newspaper takes flight down an empty street, and suddenly we find ourselves in a world made luminous with wonder. We can't summon such moments, but we can open ourselves to them when they arrive. One rainy, windy night I stand at the sink, absently washing dishes, cocooned in worry and self-doubt, when I'm startled by a movement outside the window, something dimly glimpsed through my own reflec-tion. A flicker of childhood nightmare has my heart racing: what face, toothless and grizzled, waits to press itself against the glass? I peer into the dark and see only the leaves of a begonia plant, nodding in the night breeze, their very pres-ence outside the bubble of my self-concern seeming to say, "The world is larger than your fear."

And so it is: the world itself can call us out of our preoccu-pations, our worries, our lists and agendas. In such moments our attention is arrested, quite literally stopped, and the world seems to say to us: "Don't just do something, stand there." Fear contracts, love expands. Not only our love of the world but our love of other people pulls us into larger versions of ourselves. In the midst of a busy morning, with a long list of unfinished tasks, your daughter or granddaughter asks you to bake cookies and you surprise yourself by saying yes, so that for one hour the world stops and you give yourself the gift of being fully present to her small hands, to the pleasure of her company, to sweet sticky dough. A friend asks you to sit down for a cup of coffee, and you surprise yourself by saying yes, giving yourself permission to look into another's eyes and find there exactly the thing you had been about to rush off in search of. A friend of mine once held out her hand to show me the painting that her teenage daughter had done on her thumbnail. It was the view from their dock on the lake: a sailboat in the water, an island in the distance, the sky above. I was impressed by the skill but moreso by the fact that this busy woman and her daughter had sat still together for long enough to do such a thing.

Sometimes I can sit in the meadow and simply feel the sun on me, letting this small warmth be a grace, knowing that all creation has conspired to produce this hour, this breeze lifting the hair on my forearms, this fly tickling my shin. We have all known such moments, such islands of respite. On some level we are always searching for our life's work, wanting to align our doing and our being with our highest purposes. At such moments of calm we find, to our surprise, that our life's work is here in our hands, at this very moment; it is here as we gaze into another's eyes, it is here in each breath we receive from and give back to the world.

Perhaps the art of doing nothing comes to no more than this: moments of stillness and attention, small gifts to others, most importantly the gift of our own loving presence. But I'm not sure that's enough. There *is* work to be done in the world, after all, tasks more strenuous than thumbnail painting or lounging in a chair, as difficult as it can be to do those things properly. At some point summer ends, and we return to autumn's realities. For many of us this comes as a relief. After August's compulsory laziness, we welcome September's rigor. The fall justifies and even demands our busyness: we bustle our children off to school; we pick the last tomatoes before the frost, setting the green ones to ripen on the window sill; we store window screens and worry about firewood. At our jobs the pace quickens. We're full of projects, plans, ambitions.

For us who would master the art of doing nothing, autumn brings the greatest challenge. For "doing nothing," in the way I mean it, is not literally a question of doing nothing, nor is it always a case of needing to do fewer things than we're doing now. Our challenge is to do nothing in the midst of our doing, to let our actions issue from a still center, to find within ourselves what T. S. Eliot called "the still point of the turning world."

Those who study creativity and "genius" report that the superstars of human endeavor—whether great athletes, artists, surgeons, or businesspeople—have one essential trait in common: an extraordinary ability to focus on the task at hand. The violinist practicing for hours without pause, the basketball player shooting a thousand free throws after the other players have all gone home, the deal-maker studying the numbers until dawn: each evinces a serene absorption (what the poet Donald Hall calls "absorbedness"); for each, the world vanishes and time stands still. When such a person's work involves other people, this ability to focus can be transforming for those others. The truly gifted doctors, teachers, grandmothers, managers, and leaders of all kinds make you feel, however long you're in their presence, like the most important person in the world.

But we don't have to be superstars to experience and cultivate our own moments of "absorbedness." It's a question of doing the task immediately before us as if it were our life's work. This is the sense in which I take those words from the *Tao Te Ching*: "A truly good man does nothing, yet leaves nothing undone." Nothing is left undone because when we surrender ourselves to the work of the present moment, there is nothing else to do. "A foolish man is always doing, yet much remains to be done." The foolish man is never fully present to his work but is always thinking ahead to the task that follows this one or back to tasks undone, done badly, or done well. The foolish man is always present to himself as thinking, worrying, doubting, self-congratulating, planning, regretting, and so forth, while the truly good man is always present to himself as simply doing. Or to put it more rigorously: in his non-doing the good man is present only to the doing and not to himself as an "I." For we all know those moments of calm, whether we are sipping tea, writing a memo, or driving a nail. When we give ourselves permission to do only what is immediately before us, the "I," or ego, disappears.

The Zen master Shunryu Suzuki writes that "when you do something, you should burn yourself completely, like a good bonfire, leaving no trace of yourself. . . . You should not be a smoky fire. You should burn yourself completely, with nothing remaining but ashes." So often we're caught up in the drama of our doing, making of ourselves either the virtuous hero or the suffering victim. To burn ourselves to ashes is to burn these fantasy images of ourselves, to burn the stage sets fabricated by the ego. And when we do, when we act in calm alignment with our highest purpose, we know that our actions come from beyond our small, grasping selves and issue out into a world larger than our blinkered eyes can see.

This is part of what Jesus means when he says "I have come down from heaven not to do my own will but the will of him who sent me." Throughout the Gospel of John, Jesus is pestered by people asking who he is, where he has come from, and whether he is the Messiah. "Where is your Father?" they ask him, and he answers, "You know neither me nor my Father. If you knew me, you would know my Father also." People are missing the point, Jesus is saying. They are hung up on Jesus as a man, as a personality. As Jesus the man, a Jew from Galilee, he of course does have a personality, but as Jesus the Christ he is only the vessel for his father's will. Acting in perfect alignment with that will, Jesus burns himself completely, leaving no trace. He is not, in Suzuki's terms, a smoky fire.

In Hindu terms, Jesus exemplifies the ideal of acting without karma. The way I've always heard it, by doing good actions, we accumulate good karma in order to balance bad karma we've piled up both in this life and in lives past. But my friend Cathy, the Sanskrit scholar, tells me that's mainly an American interpretation. Yes, it's better to accumulate good karma than bad, but ideally, she tells me, our actions generate no karma at all. Karma accumulates only when our actions issue from some ego, remain the work of some "I." The Hindu saint, like the Taoist sage, like Jesus, has burned his or her ego to ashes and thus perfected the art of doing nothing.

Now on many days, as autumn turns gray and cold, I would gladly trade my saintly aspirations for a small ranch within sight of New Mexico's Sangre de Cristo Mountains, where I could view snow capped peaks from a safe and sun-baked distance. Maybe I'm getting soft, but I'm skeptical of perfection. The very idea of trying for sainthood always reminds me of George Orwell's comment about Gandhi: "Saints should be judged guilty until proved innocent." Our humanness brings spice to life, and it's hard to imagine that they serve good enchiladas in heaven. Luckily, my family reminds me daily that I'm in no danger of achieving sainthood anytime soon. Most of us can count on both suffering and enjoying our humanness for the foreseeable future. That's a good thing, for the fact is, we need our humanness if we are to get closer to God. Tibetan Buddhists believe that after many lifetimes of advancement we can become a sort of temporary deity and live for a while outside human form. But to advance to ultimate enlightenment, we must return to incarnation. It's a sign of their high spiritual attainment that the deified humans welcome reincarnation, despite the suffering that human life entails. Just as Jesus needed a body in order to lay it on the cross, we need our humanness in order to become more fully divine.

These days, I'm getting plenty of practice at being human—and busy—for in the past several months I've seen my life turned inside out. Increasingly disabled, I've had to give up my college teaching career and much else. We've seen our home of nine years emptied and our worldly goods hauled here to a seasonal home now become a permanent one, as we settle in for a future where much remains unsettled. But saying that my life is in transition does no more than name what afflicts us all. For who among us does not suffer change? Though we do find our islands of calm, who among us isn't once more swept out into the storm? All our busyness, all our doing, all our works for good or ill cannot stop the whirlwind. Our hope, then, lies in learning the art of non-doing, in learning the hard truth that much of the time, as the Tao says, "The world is ruled by letting things take their course." If we lose ourselves in busyness, we may find ourselves in sitting still. If we lose ourselves in sitting still, we may find ourselves in the dance of non-doing. Let us choose to dance with Rumi, the old Sufi master, who has left us these words:

> Dance, when you're broken open.
> Dance, if you've torn the bandage off.
> Dance in the middle of the fighting.
> Dance in your blood.
> Dance, when you're perfectly free.

11

RETURNING HOME

Two nights ago, the wind was up, the first real blow of December, with 70 mile per hour gusts. At the first flicker of the lights we filled the bathtub with water, and by the time we were plunged into blackness, just after dinner, we were ready with flashlights and candles. We staggered to bed early, the kids bedded down on the living room floor by the woodstove, and we woke with big pines down across the road. This is how we dance with chaos. We change batteries and store water. We read bedtime stories to our children. We keep the chainsaw sharp, not knowing which trees or when, only that they will fall.

I'd like to think there's some value in being reminded that there's only so much we can control. I think of Robert Frost's lines:

> The tree the tempest with a crash of wood
> Throws down across our path is not to bar
> Our passage to our journey's end for good
> But just to ask us who we think we are

Lately I've been given plenty of reason to reflect on such surprises. After sticking it out as long as I could, I've finally had to give up my college teaching career in the Midwest and return for good to this one-blinking-light town in New Hampshire's White Mountains, the place of my boyhood summers, where my parents now live full-time and which in some unnamable, inner sense I have never really left. My returning home in this way is not the end of my journey—not yet—but a sudden detour. A surprise, certainly. In some ways I'm astonished at my good fortune. Who could have expected, after all, that in my early 40s I would be living a sort of gentleman's retirement in the country, with time to read philosophy, raise chickens, and supervise my children's piano practice? Each morning, I watch the sun rise, a little later and a little further south yet filling my house with light. Hoar frost glitters in the fields. My wife makes coffee, my children make their beds. Who could complain? And yet these are hardly the terms under which I had hoped to receive such a bounty. I'm in a chair with wheels. I no longer can raise my arms in joy.

But who among us gets to dictate the terms of his or her good fortune? You can't live for very long on this earth without confronting a fundamental truth: we're not in charge here, at least not entirely so. Our greatest blessings, along with our greatest burdens, seem to fall upon us unbidden. For all our planning, for all our talk of goals, for all our strategy and vision and commitment, we learn that many of our lives' most important events can't be predicted or controlled. All the plans we are in the business of making are continually being upset by both disaster and delight. How many of us could have predicted, when we first set out from our parents' homes for college or work or marriage, either our achievements or our disappointments? For how many of us has life turned out to be *exactly what we had in mind?*

All of us have at some point faced that tree fallen across the road, all of us have been forced to ask who we think we are. We have lost jobs, marriages, health. We have seen friends fail and bodies wither. With each loss the trap door opens beneath our feet and we fall, feeling the terrible wind, gazing upward at a life now forever out of reach.

Last spring, while we were packing for our move here from Illinois, I lived surrounded by boxes, seeing an entire stretch of my life hauled or thrown away. I found myself asking, "What here abides?" The home is always on some level an embodiment of the self, and mine was being emptied. In the midst of change, what lasts? Of course, traditional religion has ready answers, like this one from St. Paul: "We know that if the earthly house we live in is destroyed, we have a building from God, a house not made with hands, eternal in the heavens."

But many of us these days don't accept Paul's vision, at least not literally. Even my computer appears skeptical. Because I have trouble typing, I use speech dictation software, and when I said a house "eternal in the heavens" the words appeared on my screen as "eternal in the Hamptons." Now, some of us might prefer a house in the Hamptons to an eternity of white robes and harp lessons. And many of us doubtless find it more likely that we'll end up in the Hamptons than with the sort of house described by Paul. But even if we don't accept Paul's vision literally, still his words challenge us to imagine what home of ours *will* last. We seek continually to return home, in the face of disaster and delight, in the face of all that calls and keeps us away. We seek that sure ground of our being and our doing, the home that withstands the vagaries of time and chance and change. At the very least, we feel entitled to something more than the home Robert Frost defines mischievously as: "the place where, when you have to go there, they have to take you in."

But spiritual problems are never resolved, only transcended, and in the end we return home by recognizing that we're already there. Indeed, our true home is within. As the stoic Marcus Aurelius wrote: "Look within. Within is the fountain of good. And it will ever bubble up, if thou wilt ever

dig." Finding this fountain of goodness within us, we discover that no land is foreign; no matter where we go, we are
never strangers. We return home to the place we never left.
I know this is easier said than done. Perhaps no feeling is
more common in us than the feeling of being alone and estranged, far from the home of our fond imaginings. To some,
this is the meaning of the story of our expulsion from the
Garden of Eden. Our exile—from God, from our divine selves,
from the true nature of things, from our heart of hearts—
comes as our birthright, as the cost of our precious humanness. Feeling our estrangement, we continually yearn for
home, and each of the world's religions teaches its own way
of getting there.

This journey home is illustrated beautifully in the Old
Testament Book of Ruth. You may remember the story. In a
time of famine, Naomi leaves the Jewish homeland of Judah,
settling in Moab with her husband and two sons. Eventually
her sons marry Moabite women. Then comes Naomi's wind-
storm, her trees fallen across the road: her husband and sons
all die. Naomi, bereft and far from her people, decides to
return to her homeland, urging her daughters-in-law to "return to your mothers' houses." The daughters-in-law protest,
for they have come to love Naomi and don't want to leave
her. One of the women does eventually return to her family,
but the other, Ruth, refuses. Her words to Naomi are among
the Bible's most fondly remembered lines:

> Where you go, I will go; where you lodge, I will lodge;
> your people shall be my people, and your God my God.
> Where you die, I will die—there will I be buried.
> May the Lord do thus and so to me, and more as well,
> if even death parts me from you.

The story ends happily: Naomi and Ruth journey together
to Naomi's homeland in Judah, contrive to marry Ruth off to

Boaz, a good and wealthy kinsman of Naomi's, and at the story's end Ruth bears Naomi's first grandson, said to be the grandfather of King David (and thus, according to a later tradition, an ancestor of Jesus). It's a beautiful story of love and fidelity, of the ways new families can be formed out of misfortune. Further, Ruth's story is part of a larger development within the history told by the Hebrew Bible, which traces the evolving relationship between a people and its God. Ruth is not born a Jew but chooses to become one. Once the God of only a small desert band and one god among many in the region, the God of Abraham, Isaac, and Jacob is developing into something else altogether: the God of all creation and of all people, the home to which anyone may choose to return.

We may not believe in the personal deity that the ancient Jews believed in. For us, God may be love, the spirit of life, the creative power that works within us and in all things in every moment, our divine self, or the ground of our being. Whatever our personal concept of God—or, indeed, whatever our confusions about this subject—we can learn from Ruth's journey. Ruth is said "to return" with Naomi to Judah, but of course it is only Naomi who is actually returning. Biblical scholar Robert Alter argues that the writer of the Book of Ruth plays on the word "return" to suggest the deeper meaning of Ruth's journey. Ruth was born in Moab, and is journeying to a land she has never seen. Can we return to a place we have never been? Only if that place is within us.

Jewish history is marked by journeys: Abraham's original journey into the desert, the journey of Moses and his people out of Egypt, the Jews' return from their Babylonian exile. As this history develops, we come increasingly to understand these outward, physical journeys in terms of their inward, spiritual dimension. Ruth's story presents her as a person of character, courage, and love who meets her life's crises with steadfast faith. She has always lived close to that fountain of good within. Thus, Ruth can return home to Judah, home to God, because it's a place she has never left.

In our lives we return home again and again. Each challenge, each crisis, each dislocation gives us a chance to renew the journey. Of course, it may not seem so wonderful at the time. If I repeatedly bang my thumb with a hammer, I may not be very grateful for it, even if it gets me to improve my carpentry skills in the long run. Too often the repeated challenges and hardships of our lives seem mere repetition without advancement. We've all been through times when everything is going right: we're in the right relationship and the right job, our kids are eating their brussels sprouts, our meditations are yielding extraordinary insight and serenity. Then, wham! Down comes the hammer on the thumb, and everything we thought we were doing right goes suddenly, horribly wrong. A certain amount of this is inevitable. Life, after all, is a messy business, and there's a natural ebb and flow to the process of growing up and learning what it means to be human. Still, we'd like to think we're not going in circles.

What's needed is a structure for our spiritual life, some container to keep our growing awareness from dribbling away. As John Tarrant writes, in *The Light inside the Dark*, "Everything new needs to be held, needs a place into which it can be born." The name of this container is "character," he writes. Character, Tarrant says, is the vessel in which to hold "our swirling selves." We do not have a say in all that befalls us, but we do have a say in the shape of our own character.

Too often these days, when we hear someone speaking of the need for "character," it's a preacher or a politician wanting to impose a particular list of thou-shalt-nots on others. When I hear such talk, I'm reminded of lectures delivered by my high school's vice principal, a former pro football lineman who had redeployed his body-crushing talents toward the moral improvement of adolescents. Character, too often, is something others feel we must have beaten into us. Truth is, much of our character is under no one's control but is shaped haphazardly by our families, our communities and our culture—not to mention the genetic role of the dice by which we're made to begin with. But increasingly as we reach adulthood, we come to see character as a matter of choice. We choose practices and principles that shape our character, building either a sound vessel or a weak one. To Aristotle, for instance, choosing friends is a defining act of character, or *ethos*. We choose friends whose qualities we wish to develop or preserve in ourselves. In our daily work, in our roles as caregivers and providers, in our manner of receiving the gifts and good works of others, we can be disciplined or not, mindful or not, responsible and responsive or not, but always our actions both shape and are shaped by the vessel of character. And traditionally, religious faith and spiritual practice are thought to strengthen this vessel, creating a sound container for our developing relationship to mystery, suffering, and the Divine.

Life throws things at us that we cannot predict and cannot control. What we can control is who we are along the way. We can, like Ruth, control how much energy, compassion, and integrity we bring to our journey.

We've all heard of the sudden millionaires, the lottery winners whose lives have gone haywire. And we know others on whom success has hardened like a shell, sealing them off from friends and family. These examples teach us that it's not just bad news that carries us away from ourselves. Good fortune can threaten our integrity, too. An old Buddhist story tells of the seeker who after years of instruction and meditation goes on a pilgrimage high in the mountains, where at last he has a transforming vision that heralds his enlightenment. Full of excitement, he returns to his teacher to tell of the wonderful thing that has befallen him. The teacher, a man of many years and hard-won wisdom, replies: "Don't worry, you'll get over it." What we're after is equanimity, the poise that allows us to accept gracefully the blessings and burdens that are beyond our control. What we're after is the ability, regardless of circumstance, in the face of disappointment and happy surprise, in the face of tragedy and bliss, to return home to our true selves and our highest natures.

According to a Yiddish saying, *Mann trachts und Gött lackts:* man plans and God laughs. That doesn't mean we stop planning, even though sometimes things get pretty comic. Here's 48 hours in our household last spring: my wife and I have offered to teach summer school classes to make enough money to pay the moving van. The registrar calls to tell us we've got enough students signed up for the classes to run, and we're feeling pretty good. But then the moving company gives us an estimate $1,000 over our budget. We're cast down. That night, the phone rings: someone offers my wife part-time teaching in New Hampshire. We're raised up! The next day she gets a call back from a second person locked in a departmental war with the first: the course has been canceled, and we're once again cast into the pit. We get a second estimate on the moving: $1,000 less than the first! We break out the party hats and noise makers. Later that day the second moving guy calls back: he's made an error, and now it's $1,500 more. We eat ashes for dinner. A letter arrives in the mail: someone has insisted on paying me $1,000 for a job I said I would do for free. We sign up for hula dancing lessons. The next morning, my wife takes the car into the shop to have it checked out for our trip, and guess what? I hear God laughing.

And yet we keep on planning. How can we do otherwise? There's more at stake here than balancing our checkbooks and paying the bills. For that matter there's more at stake than our personal happiness or spiritual growth. As ethical beings we're called to improve the lives of others, our children, and our communities, a vocation that requires not simply accepting things as they are but imagining something better and working toward it.

But here's the paradox: we must strive toward goals but at the same time let them go. For as the Buddhists say, our very attachment makes us suffer. Seekers of spiritual advancement have long known the danger of wanting something too badly. The Zen Buddhist places meditation at the heart of spiritual practice, and yet Zen master Shunryu Suzuki teaches that "if our practice is only a means to attain enlightenment, there is actually no way to attain it!" In characteristic Zen fashion, Suzuki claims that "when you give up, when you no longer want something, or when you do not try to do anything special, then you do something." Equally hard on Western ears are the teachings of Lao Tzu: "When nothing is done, nothing is left undone. The world is ruled by letting things take their course."

But how can we do that? How can we do nothing when so much around us needs to be done? How can we have goals yet not grasp them too tightly? We want lives of steady purpose, lives that matter, we want to know who we are and where we're going. How can we do that while remaining open to possibility, to change, to disappointment and surprise? What might such a life look like?

I'm not sure exactly, but hitchhiking comes to mind. Anyone who has done much of it knows that hitchhiking goes best when you're not in a hurry. So I don't mean the sweaty and breathless hitchhiking you do when your car breaks down on the way to a business meeting, though I've done that kind, too. I'm thinking of the kind I did one day when I hitchhiked from Montreal back home to New Hampshire. This was another fall, another return home. I had just finished college, and I'd been traveling for five months: through the desert Southwest, up the California Coast and all the way to Seattle, then to Alaska and finally, with winter on my heels, back across Canada by train. Having spent most of the night and all of my Canadian money drinking beer and playing poker on the train, I arrived just after dawn in the heart of Montreal broke and tired and needing to get to the city outskirts. I looked at a map on the wall of the train station, took a compass reading, and started walking. Several hours later, relying on my compass and my bad high school French, I reached a place where I could hold up my cardboard sign, my destination neatly printed in black marker, and catch my first ride of the day.

Hitchhiking requires that you take what comes, that you learn to be sociable with all sorts of people, and that you be ready for delay and detour. In fact, if you're doing it in the proper spirit, there's no such thing as delay or detour. In the Tao of hitchhiking, there is no distinction between detour and the straight path, and likewise no distinction between an hour spent here or an hour spent anywhere else. This isn't to say one loses sight of the destination. A firm destination gives the journey the structure and rigor that distinguish traveling from wandering. Hence my cardboard signs, lettered neatly with the marker I carried in my pack. But you learn, when hitchhiking, not to grasp your destination too firmly, lest you miss the journey. I was continually rewriting those cardboard signs, or throwing them away. And for one stretch of the California coast, I simply held out a large piece of cardboard cut in the shape of a gigantic fist with extended thumb.

So it was fitting that, some 14 hours after walking out of Montreal, I caught the last ride of my 10,000 mile journey holding up a cardboard sign that was perfectly blank. And it was also fitting that I didn't make it home that night but got dropped off near midnight to spend the next two hours walking in the utter blackness of an untraveled country road until I lay down in a pasture, still several miles from home, aligned my body with the Milky Way, and slept until dawn.

That autumn's return proved to be one of many, and now I find myself here again, amid white pines and moonlight, twenty years older but still waiting for snow and still practicing the art of returning home.

I have a friend here in town who is a potter, and one day last summer he showed us how to make a pot. You start by slapping a lump of clay on the wheel and centering it so that it spins smoothly. To shape the clay, you press the spinning lump between your palms, gouge your thumbs into its center, and pull the whole mass toward you so the clay's rotation is no longer centered on the wheel but on the space between your hands. Squeezing between thumb and fingertips, you pull upward from base to rim, pulling the pot into form and then gently releasing it to spin smoothly on the wheel again. In a master's hands, it takes three pulls to form a pot, and the hardest part, my friend explained, is learning how to let the clay go each time. You must let go and let the clay find the center of the wheel; if you try to force it there, the pot will wobble.

This is the rhythm of our lives. We need the pulling, the striving, we need to be shaped by life. We need to be deformed so that we may return to form. For we are not angels but men and women of clay. All of us will be pulled off center, we will be shaped by both disaster and delight. So we need to learn the art of returning home, returning to center, letting go of all that binds us too tightly to both fear and to hope, letting go of our attachment to both doom and reward, letting go of all that leaves us wobbling. When we learn to return home in this way, we will return bearing gifts.

12

LIVING AT THE EDGE

I've always loved edges: the edge of night when color drains from the land, the edge of an argument where a fixed idea adjusts to other points of view, the edge of a body where skin meets air or my caress. I love edges for the vantage they provide. If you invite me to a backyard barbecue you'll see me drift away—as discreetly as one can while riding a 400-pound motorized wheelchair—to check out your property line and look for signs of history there: a broken fence, discarded tools, a change of grade where a neighbor added fill. At such edges we can see past and present together; history is made visible.

One night last spring, visiting friends northwest of Chicago, I sneaked away to the edge of their new housing development and gazed across a mile of cornfield gone fallow, waiting to sprout more driveways, lamp posts, houses, heartbreak, bliss. An alien spaceship hovered (a water tower, actually), its red lights flashing, having lowered spindly legs and a long tube to feed on the rich topsoil—10,000 years in the making—soon to be stripped off and sold for suburban lawns. A cultivator rusted in the scruff at the field's edge; the night sky glowed purple with city light; on the horizon the mountain of a landfill loomed, tongues of flame licking out of methane vents. Highway noise, distant and unstoppable, washed over all. I was seeing the beginning and ending of a world.

Here in New Hampshire the fields have suffered a different fate, taken over by woods when farmers fled this bony soil 100 years ago to work the very fields now going under subdivisions and shopping malls near Chicago and throughout the Midwest. To build our house, on land that's part of the 200-year old farm my parents own, we had to reclaim some territory from the woods, restoring what had formerly been pasture, and before that, primeval forest. The cabin where I write sits in the woods near the edge of the property, within sight of the stone wall topped with tattered barbed wire that once kept cows in but failed to stop the woods' advance once the cows had gone. From the window of my cabin I can see the shallow pit of an old farm dump, a settled heap of broken bottles and rusted cans, punctured pots and the flayed rubber soles of boots. Beyond lies the rotted, barely recognizable frame of an old truck. We stand dumbfounded before such junk, staring at the mute, recalcitrant wreck of time. The past is there before us, rusted, cracked, peeling, sinking into earth, and yet it is not there but unutterably gone, absent as the dead. You hoist a rusted bucket, its bottom reduced to rumor, an opening through which you peer at all that's vanished.

I want to think about those moments when we stand at the edge, when we feel the presence of what has gone before, when we sense the onrushing promise—or threat—of things to come. Maybe it's just the time of year. We pick our last tomatoes, not knowing they're the last until we wake one morning to see frost blanketing the fields and our petunias slumped in their beds. Trees catch fire, whole hillsides burst into flame. Armed men roam the woods; we're wakened by rifle shots. It's as if every year at this time the world imagined its own ending. Maybe, too, my interest in edges is personal. I stand at the edge of a life made shorter by illness, and can't help being pulled out of the present moment into mourning my losses, courting my fears. I sigh over my lost prowess as a hula dancer, I fear the day when I will be unable to lift a spoon of lime Jell-O to my lips.

But we all stand at the edge. The present moment is itself an edge, this evanescent sliver of time between past and future. We're called away from it continually by our earthly pleasures and concerns. Even now you may be thinking it's time for another cup of coffee and one of those blueberry muffins. Seems it's always time to be doing something other than what we're doing at the moment. While reading in your chair, you find yourself thinking about last night's argument with your spouse; you're thinking that it's time to rake leaves, check your email, get some sleep, get to work, pick up the kids, feed the boa constrictor, water the chickens, exercise the gerbils.

The present moment, like the spotted owl or the sea turtle, has become an endangered species. Yet more and more I find that dwelling in the present moment, in the face of everything that would call us out of it, is our highest spiritual discipline. More boldly, I would say that our very presentness is our salvation; the present moment, entered into fully, is our gateway to eternal life.

Now, when I say this, you could accuse me of being a mystic. And I am, but of a very ordinary kind. I don't doubt that some people throughout history, and some living today, have heard voices and seen visions. But my mysticism does not involve access to other realms, only the deeper experience of this one. Mine is the mysticism of everyday life, of the heaped laundry and the bruised toe, of overcooked broccoli and leaves spangled with dew, of sunrise and sorrow, laughter and linguine, music and mold. This everyday mysticism requires no special powers, only imagination, a doting and practiced attention to the ordinary, a willingness to be surprised by grace.

Still, when I say I'm looking for eternity in a pile of laundry you might wonder if I've been going a bit heavy on the Tabasco sauce. But I'm just being pragmatic. I don't know what, if anything, follows this life. Certain scenarios are appealing: reunion with my childhood pets, all-night jam sessions with Jerry Garcia, reincarnation as a Basset hound. But none of that may come to pass. I don't mean to discount belief in an afterlife or in reincarnation, or the comfort and moral discipline such beliefs can provide. But these are matters of faith, not knowledge in the scientific or rational sense, and as such are better left to the individual conscience. What I can know is that I am here, now, in a world of worn shoes and rose petals, seeking eternity where ever I can find it. You might say that I want my eternal life now, before it's over with.

So how to go about it? How can we cultivate this eternal present? The Buddhist practice of mindfulness, as explicated by Thich Nhat Hanh and others, offers one model. Dwelling in the moment, on our breath, on the works of our hands immediately before us, we're drawn into life's luminousness, into the mystery at the heart of ordinary things. Dwelling in the present, at least at first, involves forgetting past and future, stopping the mind's whirlwind of memory and expectation, giving ourselves a blessed hour's calm as we meditate, bake bread, walk through the forest, or play games with a child. But with further practice we may find past and future returning to our awareness, only now without bringing anxiety or distraction along with them. Instead, we become aware of living in eternity, knowing that this moment has found its proper place in the stream of all time. When we feel this way, the present moment enlarges, draws past and future into it, until we are dwelling not just in the moment but within the whole of life.

Let me give an example. Our small New Hampshire town is in love with the past, and with celebrating its own history.

Driving into the town center, with its white clapboard houses and one blinking light, you feel as though you're driving into a museum. And, mostly, that's the way we like it. The title sequence of a popular 1980s television show featured an aerial shot of the place, meant to convey to the viewer an image of classic, picturesque New England. But as a child who spent my summers there in the 1960s I sensed the lateness of the cultural hour. The fields were filling with brush, the tractors rusting, the men who used them dying or moving away. We feel the keenest nostalgia for a past we've never lived, and that's what I felt, at eight or ten years old, each time I went into our barn, with its smell of hay dust and rope, motor oil and tar. Surely this vanished world of the farm was far richer— far more real, somehow—than any world I, a kid from the suburbs, would ever know. Things we found there had a talismanic power: the cow's horn fringed with white hair, the hide folded like a blanket and stiff as wood.

Nothing cures nostalgia like growing up. I was reminded of this recently, during our annual country fair, when I rolled my wheelchair down the street after the parade of horses and oxen had gone by. Whatever its rustic pleasures may have been, our lost agrarian paradise produced a lot of manure.

Still, at our historical society museum, at the fair, or attending the Old Home Week celebration, it's easy to start feeling that the present is but a cheap copy of a more authentic past. I sit along the parade route, watching flatbed trailers roll by loaded with hay bales, corn stalks, pumpkins, and hastily costumed children being reminded to wave and smile. A bonneted and aproned girl, barely five years old and bored, drags a turkey down the street on a leash. Surely in the old days, I was thinking, people did this better. Or, because they actually lived the lives here being re-enacted, they didn't need to do these things at all. Clearly, if presentness is my goal, neither attitude—neither my boyhood nostalgia nor my adult cynicism—serves me well.

And yet at times I can escape both attitudes and see things differently. Two years ago, for instance, during our 100th annual Old Home Week, people gathered at the band stand on the fairgrounds for an "old-fashioned ice cream social." We ate ice cream and strawberry sauce out of plastic cups and did our best, I suppose, to feel old-fashioned. Then something happened, a shift from my ordinary way of seeing to what I can only call mystic vision. Suddenly it was as though I was looking at this gathering from far off, from a time 100 years in the future, when this crowd of happy people in their Gap T-shirts and Reebok shoes would be no more, would be nothing but dust and ashes, even their photographs piled into shoe boxes and forgotten in attics. From such a vantage one's generosity returns, and I saw that this moment, graced with ice cream and artificial preservatives and the ordinary talk of friends and neighbors, was as authentic as any in the town's history. From the vantage of that onlooker 100 years from now, this *was* the town's history, and we were its old timers.

My point is simple, in a way. If eternity includes all time, then we are living in eternity now. But we must widen our angle of view enough to see it. When we do, we feel in touch with life's unchanging essence, the bedrock beneath the flowing stream. We enter the eternal life beneath the surface of this passing one.

Shamans and nuclear physicists know that our limited everyday understanding of time is a result of our particular cognitive and perceptual faculties. Other forms of consciousness and thus other descriptions of reality are possible. But you don't have to beat a drum or use a particle accelerator to see multiple periods of time at once. Simply look into the heavens on a clear night. Looking at a star a 100 light-years away, you see it as it was 100 years ago. In the same moment you're seeing the more distant star next to it as it was 1,000 years ago. You're not just looking into the past but into multiple pasts. Then look into the blackness between stars (you really need a radio telescope to do this) and you can look back 15 billion years to the beginning of the universe, detecting there the residue of the big bang, a uniform background hiss reaching us from the edge of all that is.

When you're finished doing that, you're probably ready to come back to earth, where we've already got enough weirdness to keep us fully occupied. I'm reminded of the speaker of Robert Frost's poem, "Desert Places," who watches a field filling up with snow and thinks:

> They cannot scare me with their empty spaces
> Between stars—on stars where no human race is.
> I have it in me so much nearer home
> To scare myself with my own desert places.

Yes, we have plenty to scare ourselves with in this life, so this mystic vision, this living at the edge, requires an extra fearlessness. Most times, it strikes me unprepared. I can be sitting in a room full of people and eating canned peas, listening to bouzouki music, or discussing the price of ostrich futures, and suddenly I am aware that everyone in this room will one day die. It does not come to me as an idea, as something to analyze or ponder, but as a quality of vision, as though my inner cameraman had flipped on a different lens. You may accuse me of having an overactive imagination, possibly of being one slice of bread short of a sandwich. But it's more of a feeling than an actual vision. What I see does not literally change. Rather, it's as though faces, bodies, gestures have suddenly grown fluid, changeable, translucent. My awareness flickers between seeing these people as they stand here before me, solid and breathing, and sensing how the world will be when they have vanished from it.

When received in the proper spirit, such experiences are

not frightening but liberating. For in glimpsing our own transitory nature, are we not seeing a deeper truth? As the scientists tell us, we're nothing more than temporary arrangements of atoms forged in the depths of distant stars and consisting mostly of empty space. Knowing this, we discover we're both more and less important than we thought. More important because our bodies are literally made of cosmic stuff, and our being joins the dynamic, living dance of all existence. Less important because we know the cosmic dance both creates and destroys. The very particles we're made of wink in and out of being as light becomes matter and matter, light. Here science gives us new language for old truths, confirming what we've already been told by the Buddha, Heraclitus and the writers of the Psalms: the very fabric of our being glimmers and is gone; our lives are as fleeting as shadows. Knowing this, we can either despair or choose to lighten up. Jesus clearly urges the latter when with characteristic wry humor he asks, "Can any of you by worrying add a single hour to your span of life?"

When we accept our impermanence, letting go of our attachment to things as they are, we open ourselves to grace. When we can stand calmly in the face of our passing away, when we have the courage to look even into the face of a child and say, "This flower, too, will fade and be no more," when we can sense the nearness of death and feel its rightness equally with birth, then we will have crossed over to that farther shore where death can hold no fear for us, where we will know the measure of the eternal that is ours in this life.

This experience of living at the edge is not so extraordinary as it may sound. We have all had it. Perhaps you have sat with someone who was near death, and found yourself drawn into her inner radiance, into a place where pain and fear give way before a lucid awareness of the nearness of life's source. Or perhaps you have listened to a friend who has just lost a loved one, and heard in his voice, through the grief and exhaustion, a wondrous and wondering connection to life's deepest levels. Perhaps you have had it while giving birth or witnessing a birth, when we can seem to rise out of our bodies and become winged things, hovering over all we love. Or you have had it in those ordinary moments, when watching a child butter a slice of bread or a crow settle in a field, or when listening to the old nurseryman describe a hybrid azalea with the light hitting his face just so, and suddenly nothing else matters and you feel like removing your shoes and bowing down.

We all have within us this capacity for wonder, this ability to break the bonds of ordinary awareness and sense that though our lives are fleeting and transitory, we are part of something larger, eternal and unchanging.

I felt this way one day last week, when my wife and I drove into Boston to meet with my doctors at the hospital. I wasn't supposed to enjoy the day, but as it turned out, I did. On the drive down, I took in the brilliant fall colors against the blue sky. And I especially liked the chance to get out in my wheelchair in the city, rolling up and down the narrow streets of Beacon Hill. These days when I'm out in city streets I have the extra pleasure of being greeted warmly by drunkards and the homeless. I suspect that the wheelchair catches their eye, that I'm simply a spectacle, a change from the usual passersby. But I also sense they recognize me as kin, and I find I'm happy to be thus welcomed into the family of the marginal and the maimed. As my wife and I waited at one intersection for the light to change, a man staggered toward us through four lanes of traffic. He was a sight himself, with his shirt half unbuttoned and twisted sideways, his badly shaven head and bulbous red nose. He stopped short of reaching us, standing well out into the busy street, and stared. He pointed a finger at the side of his head, making a disbelieving, "Am I crazy?" gesture, and then said, "Are you guys all right?" I assured him I was. Then

I suggested he get out of the street so that he would be, too. At other times in my life, such a man would have had my defenses up. Now it seems I've less to lose and so instead could find myself moved to discover that, no matter the illness and suffering of his own life, this man's concern at that moment was for *my* welfare.

You see, we really are all in this together. There are times when the fact that we are in different bodies, or have lived in different centuries, or that some of us have died while others live on or are yet to be born, seems a trivial difference compared to what unites us and abides. Our journey takes us to suffering and sorrow, but there is a way through suffering to something like redemption, something like joy, to that larger version of ourselves that lives outside of time.

A short while after my encounter in the street, I waited outside the entrance to the hospital while my wife went to get the car. Sitting in my wheelchair in the sun, I watched people come and go. I saw people missing large pieces of their bodies, I saw people wheeled in unconscious, I saw people walking briskly while talking on cell phones, I saw families walking in bunches, shoulders bent beneath the weight of worry. An elderly couple, tiny, elegantly dressed and fragile as dried leaves, tottered toward the curb. Each held a four-point cane in one hand, and with their free hands they held onto each other, as though bracing against a wind that might any moment carry them off. On another day I might have been downcast to be part of such a scene, but now I sensed its rightness and beauty, and I felt strangely buoyant. Facing our own private calamities, we nonetheless seemed fellow travelers, carried along on the same living stream. Somehow, astonishingly, in the midst of our carnage, we had become immortal.

Some of us go willingly to the edge, some of us are driven to it, some of us find ourselves there by grace. But all of us get there at some time in our lives, when through the gateway of the present moment we glimpse something beyond. And when we do, may we open ourselves to wonder, may we surrender to the mystery that passes understanding, may we find ourselves at the threshold of this eternal life.